www.Lon[

LONGEVITY CODES

Live Longer
Stay Healthy
Remain Independent

www.LongevityCodes.com

LONGEVITY CODES

by
Fred and Tracy Herbert

LONGEVITY CODES

Copyright © 2020 by Fred Stephen Herbert and Tracy Lee Herbert

ISBN: 978-1-7351020-0-9
eISBN: 978-1-7351020-1-6

All rights reserved. No part of this book may be reproduced or transmitted in any form or by any means without written permission from the authors.

www.LongevityCodes.com

To those on a quest to live a longer, healthier, and more active life.

www.LongevityCodes.com

Disclaimer

The information found in this book is not intended as medical advice but for guidance only. Check with your medical team before making changes to diet, prescriptions, or starting an exercise program.

www.LongevityCodes.com

Table of Contents

Chapter	Title	Page
1	Foundational Approach to Longevity	1
2	Aging Paradigm Shift	8
3	Lessons from the Oldest Living People	14
4	The Motivation Factor	21
5	Prevention Principal	25
6	The 3M Formula for Longer Life	32
7	Finding the Perfect Diet	51
8	Critical Cell Signaling	60
9	Reversing Biological Age	65
10	Beat Stress for Better Health	71
11	Build a Strong Immune System	76
12	Eliminate Aches and Pains	84
13	Overcome Setbacks	93
14	The Secret to More Energy	97
15	Strategies for Better Gut Health	101
16	Taking Control of Your Health	106
17	The Master Antioxidant	110
18	Save Money While Living Longer	118
19	Move for Life	124
20	Accountability for Accelerated Results	138
21	Sleep Better and Live Longer	142
22	Supplements for Longevity	148
23	Age Slower with Longer Telomeres	158
24	Don't Go It Alone	163
25	What's Next?	167
26	References	170

"And in the end, it's not the years in your life that count; it's the life in your years."

www.LongevityCodes.com

Abraham Lincoln

"You're one choice away from a longer and healthier life!"
Tracy Herbert

www.LongevityCodes.com

Introduction

Welcome to Longevity Codes!

Years ago, we backpacked to the bottom of the Grand Canyon. That's a grueling 10-and-a-half-mile hike that drops over one mile in elevation. We met a vibrant and energetic couple at the bottom and was shocked when we discovered he was 86, and she was 84 years old. This couple hikes this strenuous trek to the bottom and back to the top twice a year. This inspirational couple has been our role model ever since. When we get off track, we quickly return to think of them and how we want to be just like them as we get older.

This book is for those wanting to find the codes, keys, and principles needed to live a longer, healthier, and more active life. This quest is for adding extra years while making those years healthy, fulfilling, and productive.

Tracy was diagnosed with a chronic, life-threatening disease over 40 years ago, and the medical experts all agreed she'd be dead within 20 years and die with horrible complications.

After leaving the hospital at the age of 17, she was on a mission to prove these doctors wrong, started researching at a college medical library, and continues studying today.

Meeting "Gina" changed Tracy's life. This single mom was desperate to lose weight and was struggling to pay the bills, and her doctor told her she had prediabetes. The two started meeting at the local school track. Once Gina began to see results, she was thrilled, and her confidence quickly grew. With Tracy's love of fitness, health, and wellness, she decided to become a Certified Personal Trainer. Using those

www.LongevityCodes.com

skills in addition to being a trained wellness coach, and her psychology degree, Tracy started coaching and hasn't stopped since. These experiences, combined with living with Type 1 diabetes, brought Tracy to the realization that she wanted to dedicate her life to help others live longer and healthier.

To "celebrate" the 40th anniversary of her diagnosis at the age of 57, Tracy completed a solo 3,527-mile bicycle ride from San Francisco to New York City. She proved her health and wellness strategies work by this epic feat and provided hope and encouragement to others facing difficult challenges.

Fred's motivation for getting healthy started much differently. His nickname was "supplement junkie" because he took every supplement known to man. He was always looking for a magical quick fix. When they married, he was on multiple prescriptions, overweight, and on our first bicycle ride together about passed out after a mile. He wouldn't listen and didn't need or want a health coach, especially his wife. After several years had passed, and his health continued to decline, he was ready for a change.

Now, he's off all medications, can ride his bicycle 50 miles, at a healthy weight, and Fred feels stronger and healthier than he can remember. What's even better is he's in his mid-60's and working on an epic adventure that will push him to the extremes.

Fred and Tracy are on a quest to help others achieve their health and wellness goals, just like they have.

www.LongevityCodes.com

Chapter 1
Foundational Approach to Longevity

In 2004 this journey began. After enjoying several days of recuperating and hiking around the bottom of the Grand Canyon, it was time to prepare for the hike out. Backpacking the Grand Canyon is a grueling 10 ½ mile downhill trek carrying a 35-pound pack and dropping over 5,000 feet in elevation, makes even the fittest endurance athlete take notice, but not our role models. While preparing to hike out, we met an 86 and 84-year-old couple who do this adventure twice a year. We were amazed at their fitness level and zest for life. This encounter changed our lives, gave us hope, and they've been our role models ever since. Meeting them was a mindset change and fueled our desire to be just like them in our 80s and beyond.

These foundational eight concepts are required to have the right mindset for longevity. Take time to digest these and evaluate where you are on your journey.

Core Concept #1 – You are responsible

You must accept full responsibility for your current and future health. What's the status of your physical and mental health? It's never too late to take control! Realizing and accepting full responsibility for your current state will drive your ability to make the necessary changes to improve the future. Once you know, you are in the driver's seat, and not a victim of circumstances, it empowers you to make the necessary changes. Forces like family, friends, society, doctors, and temptations, can get in the way, but you cannot blame them. That gives them the power and not you.

At the age of 17, Tracy had that moment after being diagnosed with Juvenile Diabetes referred to now as Type 1 Diabetes. This type of diabetes is an autoimmune disease that cannot be prevented, and there is no known cure. Type 2 Diabetes is the most common; approximately 95% of those with diabetes have this type, and it's believed to be lifestyle-related. After a few months of living in fear and desperation, she said to herself, "Tracy, you can be bitter or better, what are you going to choose?" She chose better and has lived with this chronic disease for over 40 years. Because of her drive to be a success and not a statistic, she became a diabetes advocate and a health and wellness coach. And at the age of 57, she completed a solo 3,527-mile bicycle ride across the United States to spread awareness and hope. She took responsibility for her health and has outlived her life expectancy by over 20 years.

When you decide that you are responsible, your life will change!

Core Concept #2 – Age is just a number

The Bible says, "As a man thinks in his heart, so is he." If you think you are old, you're right! You look, act, and feel the way you think. Stop and think for a second, isn't this true? Remember the couple mentioned earlier in this chapter that we met at the bottom of the Grand Canyon, who was 86 and 84 years old? This couple didn't let their age stop them from having an active life. Neither should you.

www.LongevityCodes.com

The expectations of aging that your grandparents had are no longer valid. Let's change the view by believing what is possible. Charles Eugster is a great example because he smashed the sprint records at the age of 96. What about the 100-year old yoga teacher Tao Porchon-Lynch who says, "Age can never hope to win while your heart is young?" Or Dorian "Doc" Paskowitz, who was still surfing every day at the age of 90. Growing up, Jack LaLane was a prominent figure in our home. No, he didn't live there but was always on TV. He was considered the Godfather of Fitness and well known for his feats of strength by swimming and towing boats in his 80s and lived a robust and healthy life until 96. Don't you want to have a story like theirs?

Like our friends at the bottom of the Grand Canyon, find good role models and realize you can take control and live an active life in your 90's and beyond.

Core Concept #3 – Have a future focus

What's your big, "Why?" Goals and dreams for the future are paramount for living a longer, healthier life. Knowing your "Why" for living a longer, healthier, and active life is essential for being fulfilled and taking the actions required to achieve that goal. When you don't have a compelling "Why," you won't make the daily decisions needed to accomplish it. Small daily changes add up to significant results over time.

Adolph Zukor, the founder of Paramount Pictures, approaching his hundredth birthday, said, "If I'd known how old I was going to be, I'd have taken better care of myself." That is funny but so true. How many people are living their last few decades with poor physical and mental health?

Wishing they would have done things differently regarding their health choices, doesn't work. Don't let that be you! That is what this book is all about—helping you get the most out of life.

Core Concept #4 – Health starts at the cellular level

50 to 70 trillion cells reside in the human body. These cells continuously die and replace themselves. Most diseases occur when cells become damaged. Fifty million cells die daily, and the focus on eating healthy is about giving cells the building blocks needed to repair and rebuild healthy cells. Future chapters will dive deeper into the process of how to improve the cells ability to communicate, repair, and replace.

Everything you consume impacts the health of your cells. Aging is all about keeping your cells healthy and winning the battle against oxidative stress.

Core Concept #5 – Education must be a priority

Information and education help you make the right choices when it comes to health and longevity. That's what this book is all about—providing information that enables you to pursue your goal of living a longer and healthier life.

Health information is continually changing. A good example is the war on fat and that all fat was unhealthy. Discovered years later, the sugar industry funded the study that promoted this revolution. Decades later, it has proven that not all fats are unhealthy or cause heart disease. Still, new research is showing the culprit is sugar. The Low-Fat Revolution made people heavy and unhealthy. The mainstream health system is not always the best place to get an education.

This book provides the latest scientific research and information to help you decipher fact from fiction.

Core Concept #6 – Take action

Today you have lots of information about how to be healthy, but when you do not put it in to practice, you will fail. You know what you should be doing, so why aren't you doing it?

The key is to act on what you already know. This book provides additional information with the latest research on living a longer, healthier life. For this book to be valuable to you, you must act on what you are learning and apply it!

Be willing to act NOW!

Core Concept #7 – My medical team doesn't always know best

In the United States, the system is focused on fixing symptoms and not getting to the root cause. Many physicians today are receiving training from the pharmaceutical industry. When a physician leaves medical school, their education is already outdated. The pharmaceutical companies are right there to help treat you with the latest medicine to fix all your problems.

It's not all the physician's fault. Most patients ask the physician to prescribe something to make the problem go away. When the doctor dares to tell you to quit smoking, drink less alcohol, eat better, eat less, and get out and exercise more, you might be appalled. Many patients say, "Doc, you don't understand; it's too hard." When patients do not take appropriate action, what is the doctor to do, he or she must treat the symptoms.

The United States health system is upside down. Let's put more energy into preventing disease instead of treating the disease when it rears its ugly head.

Core Concept #8 – If possible, start with natural approaches

The blame is not all on the pharmaceutical companies; patients must take responsibility. Most people want the quick, easy fix. The doctor says, "Joe, you need to cut back on sugar and salt," and Joe says, "can't you just give me a pill for that?" Consider alternative solutions to avoid this problem.

Here's an example: Tracy went to the doctor and was concerned that her blood pressure had crept up. Instantly the doctor prescribed blood pressure medication. After talking with her doctor and pharmacist, she decided to look for a natural approach. While researching, Tracy found that unfiltered fermented beet juice is as effective as most blood pressure medication and started drinking it daily. On the next trip to the doctor's office, her physician was shocked that her blood pressure was in range. She proceeded to tell the doctor the story of researching for natural approaches and found drinking beet juice was the best choice for her. The physician had not heard this strategy before and immediately went to her computer and found supporting scientific research. To the doctor's credit, she said she would tell her patients to try this approach first.

www.LongevityCodes.com

Remember core concept #1. You are responsible!

As you continue to read, you'll learn how to take control of your health at a cellular level and provide your body with the tools needed to live a longer, healthier life.

Get additional FREE RESOURCES at
www.LongevityCodes.com

Chapter 2
Aging Paradigm Shift

Living a longer and healthier life requires a shift in thinking or a change in our paradigm. Having a paradigm shift means you must change your views and attitudes about aging along with your self-talk.

Have you ever talked with a group of friends who complain about turning older? The same thing happened to us. During a recent gathering with friends around our age, the conversation quickly turned to complaining about their aches and pains and getting older. They had given up on the idea of being healthy, leading an active life, and felt destined to a sedentary life. While we are the same age, we refuse to allow ourselves that kind of thinking. On the drive home that evening, we discussed how desperately they needed a change of mind, along with the concepts in this book.

As mentioned in the previous chapter, our view of aging changed when we met the 86 and 84-year-old couple at the bottom of the Grand Canyon. After the conversation with our friends, and remembering our role models, we knew something needed to change. It was at that point we realized this book was required to help others recognize the importance of having their mindset radically changed. Doesn't everyone want to live a longer and healthier life?

What is your view of aging?

Do you see yourself in your 80's and 90's being the most productive and rewarding time of your life? Or do you live in constant fear of those years living in a downhill spiral of poor health accompanied by physical and mental decline?

That's not us!

Here are four ways to change the belief on aging:

1. Get rid of negative views of aging.
2. Understand you are in control.
3. When you surround yourself with positive active role models that prove this is possible, you begin to believe it.
4. Apply the strategies in this book and see the impact it has on your life.

> *"We don't stop playing because we grow old; we grow old because we stop playing."*
> George Bernard Shaw

Remove Negative Views of Aging

Thanks to advances in healthcare, technology, and lifestyle changes, people are living much longer. In the 1950s, the average life expectancy of a man in the United States was 67 and 73 for a woman. Today the life expectancy for men is 76 and 81 for a woman. Experts predict that by 2030 the average age for men will be just under 80 and a little over 83 for women. That number should continue to climb. These statics are the first reason to change your view on the potential of what your life expectancy could be. Each year technology improves the chance for you to live longer. When you realize this is possible, you will implement the strategies in this book.

Another reason why it is essential to change your views about living longer is due to the increase in centenarians living today. Centenarians are people 100 years old and older. According to The United Nations report on World Population Prospects[1], life expectancy worldwide has increased eight years from 1990 to 72.6 years in 2019. By 2050 it's expected to increase to 77.1. The world population of centenarians was 95,000 in 1990, 451,000 in 2015, and projected to climb to 3,676,000 by the year 2050.

The number of centenarians is increasing yearly, which means statistically, you could be one too. Therefore, you should be taking steps now to improve your health so that those last decades will be exciting, meaningful, and fulfilling. Changing your mindset is the first step to living a longer, more enjoyable life.

People who live the longest achieved it without the current research associated with longevity. Armed with the information found in this book, along with new research, and technology, you are on a course to live much longer. More people will be breaking records for living the longest than the current centenarians. By now, the light bulb is going off, and you realize that living to 120 and beyond is within reach.

That's what this book is all about. Each chapter contains strategies proven to help you live a longer and healthier life. We are on this journey, just like you!

Keep reading and TAKE ACTION on the strategies found in this book!

Surround yourself with people who have the right mindset!

Want a great way to change your mindset? Fred had a significant change in his mindset by going to 5K and 10K walks/runs and seeing the number of participants in their 70's, 80's, and 90's still running and competing. Since Tracy has been running and competing in long-distance bicycle rides for decades, she knew this to be accurate. She was happy when the light bulb finally went off for Fred.

Think you cannot be physically active at an older age? Here are athletes from around the world, proving age is just a number. Look at these World Records[2]:

- 100-meter dash World Record is held by Fauja Singh from the United Kingdom with a time of 23.40 seconds at the age of 100
- Fauja Singh also has the record in the 100-age group for the 200 meters, 400 meters, 800 meters, 1500 meters, mile, 3000 meters, 5000 meters, and the marathon.
- 80-meter hurdles Ralph Maxwell from the United States holds world Record in the 90-year-old bracket with a time of 21.62 at the age of 91.
- Ralph Maxwell has the 200-meter hurdle record at the age of 90
- Donald Pellmann from the United States at the age of 100 holds the World record in the Long Jump.
- Julia Hawkins for the United States holds the World record for the 100 meters at the age of 101.
- Betty Jean McHough of Canada holds the Women's 90-95 bracket record in the marathon in just over 7:03:59.
- How about Olga Kotelko from Canada who took up track at the age of 77. She has 30 world records and more than 750 gold medals and was still winning World Masters Athletics Championships at the age of 95.

www.LongevityCodes.com

> *"I think your age is just a number. It's not your birthday; it's how you age, which makes the difference."*
> Olga Kotelko

Living longer and healthier requires having the right mindset. Here are a few tips to get you started and keep you motivated:

- Mindsets are not carved in stone and can be changed.
- Influences by family, friends, culture, where you live, and the environment impacts your mindset. Please do not underestimate the power this has on you.
- Approximately 80% of the 12,000 to 60,000 thoughts per day are negative! Replacing negative thoughts with positive ones will improve your overall health and happiness.
- Winston Churchill said, "comparison is the thief of joy." Be cautious not to allow social media to fuel negativity, especially with comparison.
- Self-talk can be either positive or negative; choosing positive thoughts is critical!

When thinking positively, even having subliminal reminders help you remember that aging can be a wonderful, fulfilling, and the best time of your life. Having this mindset will help you feel younger, empowered, and strong.

As Tracy always says:

"We All Have Two Choices!"

Apply this quote to your attitude about aging.

www.LongevityCodes.com

One Choice: Take a pessimistic view of aging, take no action, and live the rest of your life with little or no control over your health and longevity.

--- or ---

Better Choice: Have an optimistic view of aging, realize you can take control of your health, and live life to the fullest. You would not be reading this book if this was not you.

Let's make a paradigm shift NOW and take the positive, optimistic view of aging!

Chapter 3
Lessons from the Oldest Living People

Researchers have been studying for years areas of the world where people live to 100 and beyond at rates higher than the United States, except for Loma Linda, California. These regions are Okinawa (Japan), Sardinia (Italy), Nicoya (Costa Rica), Icaria (Greece), and the Seventh-day Adventists living in Loma Linda, California.

The longest living people have these eight strategies in common:

Have a Purpose

You must KNOW your "WHY"? When you have a clear **purpose**, you will make the choices necessary to reach your longevity goals. If you're like us, you have more things to do, learn, places to go and see, then you can accomplish. To have mental clarity and physical health in your 70's, 80's, and beyond, you need a purpose now that is so strong it makes you want to get out of bed and achieve it. Having a purpose is shown to add seven years to your life according to several research studies. Want to recover faster, lower blood pressure, reduce stress, and have improved surgical outcomes? Have a purpose! What a sad way to end the last few decades without a sense of purpose. Not us! Knowing your "WHY" is critical for longevity and good health!

Be Physically Active

People who live the longest move naturally and get plenty of physical activity, and don't lift weights, join expensive gyms or run long distances. In Ikaria, Greece, the poor live the longest, which is contrary to what you might think. The reason could be because they live high in the mountains, and walking to their neighbors can be a strenuous activity. They also spend more time outside gardening. Another example is New York City residents live almost three years longer than the rest of the United States. Is it because they have less stress? No, of course not. If you've ever been to New York City, you've noticed that they walk everywhere and fast. Is this a contributing factor? Walking is easy and a great way to get natural movement. As you age, it is vital to maintain your flexibility, and being active has helped countless centenarians stay healthy. Following their strategies is a reminder for everyone to find natural ways to move throughout the day.

Learn to Relax

The longest living people have this in common; they find ways to reduce stress. Chronic stress leads to many health issues like:

- Digestive issues
- Heart disease
- Chronic Headaches
- Weight gain
- Depression and Anxiety
- Trouble Sleeping
- Concentration and Memory Problems

<www.LongevityCodes.com>

Each region reduces stress in different ways. In Ikara, Greece, for example, they reduce stress with activities like napping, the Seventh-day Adventists pray, and the Okinawans **spend time daily remembering their ancestors. In Sardinia, they** enjoy happy hour with friends and family. How do you reduce stress? Stop for just a minute, and think about what works best for you. If you find it challenging to de-stress, here are some recommendations:

- It's hard to be stressed when you are physically active. The act of moving and doing something physical melts away stress.
- You may not get enough oxygen, so try deep breathing. Many folks breathe just enough to keep from passing out. Learning deep breathing exercises will make a big difference in how you handle stress.
- Eat Better and ask yourself if your diet is contributing to the problem.
- Slowing down and learning to say no helps you evaluate and see if there's too much on your plate.
- One of the best ways to reduce stress is to get out in nature, and it does for us.
- Learn a new hobby or spend time on your old hobbies.
- Get enough sleep!
- Learn relaxation techniques like meditation.
- If stress becomes overwhelming, talk to someone. Saying it out loud helps.
- Are you putting too much stress and pressure on yourself? Give yourself grace as you do for others.
- Find and eliminate personal stress triggers.
- Avoid too much caffeine, alcohol, and nicotine.

Don't Overeat

Eat a smaller amount to live longer! The people around the world who live the longest do not eat like individuals in the United States. When our son Josh left Japan, returning to the United States, he was shocked by the portion size compared to what he was used to in Japan. A good rule of thumb is adopting the practice to stop eating when you feel 80% full. It's simple; those people who live the longest use this tool, and it works for them. If you think you've consumed enough food but are still hungry, wait 20 minutes to see how you feel. Using this tool coincides with the longest living people on the planet and helps tremendously with weight loss. Another tool that studies have proven works is to use smaller plates because you eat less, and it tricks your mind to think that you have had enough to eat. Scientists have recognized the connection between eating less and longevity.

Less Meat More Plants

Those who live the longest eat meat on average five times or less a month. Most Centenarians studied, ate an abundance of beans, lentils, fish, fruits, and vegetables. We enjoy a good steak like many of you, but this is interesting. Meat is high in saturated fat and raises your bad LDL cholesterol. Researchers suggest that the more red meat eaten, the higher the risk of developing colorectal cancer. The more sugar and processed foods consumed creates an increased risk of developing heart disease and certain types of cancer. Like those that live to 100 and more, you need to stay away from processed foods as much as possible, cook at home more to control the quality of food, and eat more veggies. When they eat meat, they only eat about 3-4 ounces at a time, which is about the size of a deck of cards. For longevity, consider cutting back on meat as we have.

Faith

Participating in a faith-based setting helps you live longer. Of the 263 centenarians studied[1], only five did not belong to a community of faith-based people. For longevity, it didn't matter the type of religion or denomination attended, but if you want to live longer than the average person, get involved in a faith community. Attending four times a month can add four to 14 extra years of life. The National Institute of Health found benefits for those who actively participate in faith-based gatherings. Participants showed lower levels of depression, smoked less, and have friends who believe the way they do, compared to those who do not attend. Frequently practicing meditation and prayer is found to help reduce stress and lowers issues with anger.

Close Family Connections

The people living the longest had their aging parents near them; their children and grandchildren also lived close. Those with life partners were able to add another three years for longevity. Harvard Health[2] reported in a study of 127,545 American's, the married men were healthier than men who had never been married or who were divorced or widowed. Another benefit found people in committed relationships were less lonely and had stronger social support. A Japanese study found men who never married were three times more likely to die from heart disease than men who were married. The intent is not to make you feel bad if you are not married or in a serious relationship, because having friends and strong social support helps bridge the gap. Finding encouraging people who help you through life's journey is critical for good health and longevity.

Strong Social Connections

Having a robust and healthy support system is critical for good health. A study[3] found that exceptional social support helped people reduce depression. The study also proved they have a lower risk of smoking, and believe it or not, when you have a good group of friends, you are less likely to be obese.

"In poverty and other misfortunes of life, true friends are a sure refuge. They keep the young out of mischief; they comfort and aid the old in their weakness, and they incite those in the prime of life to noble deeds."
Aristotle

Good friends are there to celebrate the good times in your life and will also be there with a shoulder to cry on in bad times. The better friendships you have as you age, the longer you will live. Without friends, you have a higher risk of developing diabetes, heart disease, and depression in your golden years. Do you have a friend in your life who will call or text you at 5:30 in the morning to remind you to work out? What about the friend who cheers for you when you lose weight, or start to eat healthier? Friendship is essential, but you need friends who are like-minded and ready to walk through all phases of life with you. Call a friend today and tell them how much they mean to you. It will make their day and is excellent for your health.

www.LongevityCodes.com

The eight areas covered, which are typical for the longest living people around the world, might seem a bit of a challenge. Look at each of these and determine where your most significant gaps are and start working on them today. Over time, you can incorporate all these into your daily life.

"Generally speaking, there are two kinds of learning: experience, which is gained from your own mistakes, and wisdom, which is learned from the mistakes of others."
John C. Maxwell

Get additional FREE RESOURCES at
www.LongevityCodes.com

Chapter 4

The Motivation Factor

"Wanting something is not enough. You must hunger for it. Your motivation must be compelling to overcome the obstacles that will invariably come your way."
Les Brown

Do you find it a challenge to stay motivated?

Find what motivates you! The best way to do it is to project the current behavior and visualize how it impacts the future.

Have you ever declared that today would be the day to change a negative behavior and found yourself quickly going back to the old way? If you're like us, you're probably nodding your head up and down.

Anyone who has ever decided they were going to get healthy, eat right, and exercise, has experienced setbacks.

Weight loss is a typical example that many have struggled with from time to time. According to the Center for Disease Control (CDC)[1], 71.6% of Americans are either overweight or obese.

Something must change! Of the millions of those struggling with being overweight or obese, most probably have tried staying motivated at some point. But eventually, you return to your unhealthy lifestyle because of not having the right system in place to keep you motivated.

www.LongevityCodes.com

The secret we are sharing is not a secret because you'll recognize it immediately as being the truth.

Remember Ebenezer Scrooge from Charles Dickens book "A Christmas Carol?" The secret to motivation in your health journey is in this story.

What motivated Scrooge to transform his life? It was the Ghost of Christmas Future. When the last ghost exposed Scrooge to his future, everything changed. It was what he needed at that moment to change his life and improve his future.

Here's the secret.

Let's call it the "Scrooge Effect."

PROJECT INTO THE FUTURE!

That's right! You must realistically look at how current behaviors impact the future.

The challenge lies in the difficulty of looking at the truth about your current behavior. And scare tactics seldom work, but they do for some. What scared and motivated Tracy, when she was diagnosed with Type 1 diabetes over 40 years ago, was seeing pictures of people who had their legs amputated due to diabetes complications. We all tend to think, "It won't happen to me," but in her case, she used it as a motivating factor.

Several years ago, when a family member was in the cardiac ICU unit of the hospital, almost every patient in that area was overweight and had diabetes. Both of which possibly contributed to their life-threatening heart issues. They all likely wished they had made better choices earlier in life.

You do not want to wake up in the hospital tomorrow with a heart attack. Do something today to improve your health!

"Insanity is doing the same thing over and over again and expecting different results."
Albert Einstein

Do not fall into this way of thinking!

Deep down, you know the changes needed but struggle with the motivation to do it.

Here is a visualization exercise that helps. Find a quiet place and think about the future impact of your current behaviors. Like Scrooge, see the future and all its negative consequences as clearly as possible. Make it real! Make it terrible! Make it scary enough that you will do whatever it takes to keep that from being your future. It's like time travel; you have the opportunity right now to have your future self tell you what you should be doing.

Do not stay stuck with behaviors that keep you unhealthy. For example, overeating, eating the wrong things, drinking calorie-laden beverages, being a couch potato, lack of sleep, stress, worry controlling your thoughts, and the list goes on. The compound effects of these unhealthy habits will impact your future. Your future self will thank you for the changes you make today.

Find what motivates you, whether positive or negative, and use it!

Here is another strategy if you struggle with motivation. Most successful people have coaches who help them along the way. Tracy's coaching clients find value in her helping

www.LongevityCodes.com

them stay motivated to make better health choices consistently. Day in and day out can be challenging, but having someone alongside supporting you makes a big difference. It's easy to slide back into your old habits. If you find yourself slipping back, remember the Scrooge Effect and don't allow your future to be grim.

Check out
LONGEVITY CODES COACHING PROGRAM
www.LongevityCodes.com
Our **Longevity Codes Certified Coach** will help you implement the principles in this book and provide the tools and accountability you need to achieve fast results.

www.LongevityCodes.com

Chapter 5

Prevention Principal

"An ounce of prevention is worth a pound of cure."
Benjamin Franklin

After speaking at an event on prevention, taking control of health, and overcoming setbacks, an attendee reached out to Tracy for additional help. During one of the coaching sessions, he revealed his struggle of being diagnosed with prediabetes and felt hopeless. After several months of using strategies she laid out for him, his doctor was amazed at his progress. And the best news his blood test results deemed him no longer prediabetic.

This code is straightforward.

AVOID DISEASE!

Another client wasn't so lucky. He had Type 2 diabetes for over a decade. During our first strategy session, he revealed that his doctor never told him to get his blood sugars under control. Although this is hard to imagine, he consistently had blood glucose readings in the 300 to 400 range. It didn't affect his daily life; he never felt bad, so he didn't do anything about it. Now he's fighting severe diabetes-related eye complications because of all those years of high blood sugars, which leads us back to one of the core principles of this book. Be responsible for your health, and even if you cannot see or feel it, you must understand what is happening in your body at a cellular level.

Thinking it will not happen to me is common. The smoker knows the long-term damage of cigarettes. Still, its harmful effects are slow and invisible until it too late. Similarly, the alcoholic cannot see or feel the damage to the liver until it's too late.

How about the other side of this equation?

Why don't people apply health strategies daily that they know will prevent disease? The same thing applies here; individuals do not always feel or see the results, so they stop taking the preventive action.

Why isn't society eating more organic foods? Research shows that eating organic does improve longevity because of the reduced toxins. Approximately 30% of U.S. households purchase some organic foods. Of that number, probably only a small percentage are eating only organic. Why do so few people eat organic foods which have more nutrients, less pesticides, chemicals, and are plain healthier? It is a great prevention strategy, but you do not feel any different. You may not be able to pinpoint why you feel so healthy, but this strategy might prevent some horrific health issues caused by toxic foods.

Years of applying these prevention strategies have helped Fred stay healthy and medication-free through his mid-sixties. Going for a 25-mile bicycle ride is no problem, and his next goal is completing a century bicycle ride (100 miles). The distance of this bicycle ride is not to brag, but to provide hope. Still, we have been researching and practicing these strategies for years and guarantee they work.

www.LongevityCodes.com

Tracy is another example of applying these strategies to overcome setbacks. She has lived with Type 1 diabetes for over 42 years with no complications. Doctors told her she would die within 20 years, have horrible diabetes-related complications, and never be able to have children. She proved every medical expert wrong when this grandmother completed a solo 3,527-mile bicycle ride across the United States starting in San Francisco and finishing in New York City. When asked how she accomplished this amazing feat, she always credits her 3-M Formula. Learn more about the 3-M Formula in the next chapter.

Supplements are another approach to prevention! More in-depth information on supplements is covered later in Chapter 11, but these six are critical for longevity:

- Vitamin C
- Magnesium
- Redox Signaling Molecules
- Polyphenols including Resveratrol
- Probiotics
- Vitamin D

The main reason to supplement is to give your cells everything needed to be healthy. Even though you may not feel the positive effects immediately, when purchasing high-quality supplements, research has proven that they support a longer, healthier life.

Only 25% of Americans take Vitamin C supplements even though it is known to be a powerhouse antioxidant, boosts immunity, protects memory, and fights heart disease risk factors. Why only 25%? The answer is clear, if you start taking Vitamin C for a few months and don't feel any positive effect, you decide why bother. This same thing

www.LongevityCodes.com

applies to any of these valuable six supplements or choosing healthy food options.

If you're like Tracy, who once believed vitamins and supplements didn't work, she recommends you look at the research and the quality of the supplements. She is now a strong advocate for supplementing in addition to eating healthy. There is a whole science around the best time to take a supplement, the best form to take, the best dose, and to take with food if necessary. The Recommended Daily Allowance (RDA) is the minimum dose needed to avoid major health issues. But more is not always best, follow the advice from your physician and read the directions carefully.

Magnesium is another nutrient needed for good health. Magnesium is known to help regulate blood sugar, lower systolic blood pressure while helping muscles to relax, just to name a few of the benefits. If you decide that supplementing is right for you, do not waste money on inferior products, because you may not receive any benefits.

- Epsom salt is also known as magnesium sulfate, which helps to relax muscles and detox.
- Magnesium malate is useful for improving energy and helps with muscle soreness.
- Magnesium threonate supports memory and brain health.
- Magnesium chloride is often used in a spray and absorbs well on your skin.
- Magnesium citrate helps with relaxation.
- Magnesium glycinate could help improve sleep.
- Magnesium oxide can help treat constipation.

See what we mean? This example with magnesium is also typical with other supplements. Do your research and make sure to focus on quality. Most of the time, the higher quality products cost more because the manufacturers have the research backing it up, along with using superior ingredients. But is it truly more expensive? How costly is poor health? Waking up in the ICU is never cheap, and neither is an adverse health diagnosis.

You've heard it before!

"Health starts at a cellular level."

Here's what we do for our cellular health:

We supplement daily with redox signaling molecules to help our cells communicate, repair, and regenerate. To learn more visit: www.LongevityCodes.com/redox

Next, we take a high-quality multi-vitamin. Even though we spend more, as we mentioned earlier, it's not a waste of money. We have found a big difference and understand it is best for our future.

Powdered polyphenol extract is another supplement in preventing oxidative stress. It is full of superfruits like mulberries, blackberries, cranberries, blueberries, and the list goes on. Why do we add this to our supplement toolbox? Because it's challenging to get the right amount of these essential nutrients in our daily diet, and this form won't spike Tracy's blood sugar.

Probiotics is another tool that helps with longevity and strengthening the immune system. Experts call the gut "the second brain" because many of our health systems have a gut connection.

Vitamin D is another vital supplement because most American's are deficient in this crucial vitamin. Sunshine is the best way, but overexposure to the sun can cause skin damage and certain cancers. Having your Vitamin D levels checked is an essential strategy.

The aging process is primarily due to the cellular damage caused by oxidative stress. The method of either improving or damaging cells happen slowly and is usually not noticeable. Tracy will tell you she feels better and has more energy than she did in her mid-thirties, and she does. It is possible for you too. Don't give up!

Prevention is a longevity key. People practice daily prevention strategies.

- Why wear a seatbelt? Prevention
- Why have a smoke detector? Prevention
- Why have an annual physical? Prevention
- Why not smoke? Prevention Right!
- Why do we eat healthy? Prevention

Just like you, we're trying to be more intentional! You must be all in and not look back and wonder what happened.

The CDC[1] estimates that eliminating three risk factors– poor diet, inactivity, and smoking – would prevent: 80% of heart disease and strokes, 80% of type 2 diabetes, and 40% of cancers. The CDC says that six out of ten adults in the United States have a chronic disease, and four out of ten have two or more chronic conditions.

What prevention strategies are you focusing on for longevity?

Focusing on prevention helps us live more years, and the last few years will be more active and fulfilling.

www.LongevityCodes.com

It's a known fact that the health system in the United States is not prevention-focused, but instead, treatment concentrated. The pharmaceutical companies research drugs to treat disease, not ways to prevent it.

> *"I have argued for years that we do not have a health care system in America. We have a disease-management system."*
> Andrew Weil, M.D.[2]

Dr. Weil is right! Taking control of your health and not relying on the healthcare system is paramount for good health and longevity.

By reading this book, you have already proven that you are the kind of person who is looking for better health and a longer, more fulfilling life.

Place sticky notes on your mirror, in the office, car, refrigerator, and other places and write the word "Prevention" on it. Using this approach reminds you of the commitment you've made to yourself for a longer and healthier life.

You are already practicing some of the prevention strategies in this book. Keep it up! Don't quit because you don't see immediate results. Trust the process because it takes time and will pay high dividends in the long run. Failure to do so will have devastating consequences on your health and quality of life.

Good health is an investment, and your future self will thank you for it. Every dollar spent on improving health is a down-payment for a healthier tomorrow.

Chapter 6

The 3M Formula for Longer Life

After being diagnosed with Type 1 diabetes at the age of 17, Tracy started working on strategies for living healthy despite diabetes. This Formula is her key for outliving her life expectancy and living healthy with diabetes with no complications. Tracy's 3M Formula is the culmination of over 40 years of research and application of these strategies for herself and her clients.

In the image below, the Mind is the most significant cog because it is the first and foremost critical step for change. Once the mind adapts, then eating and exercise will quickly follow. Together the three gears are synergistic and vital for living a longer, healthier life.

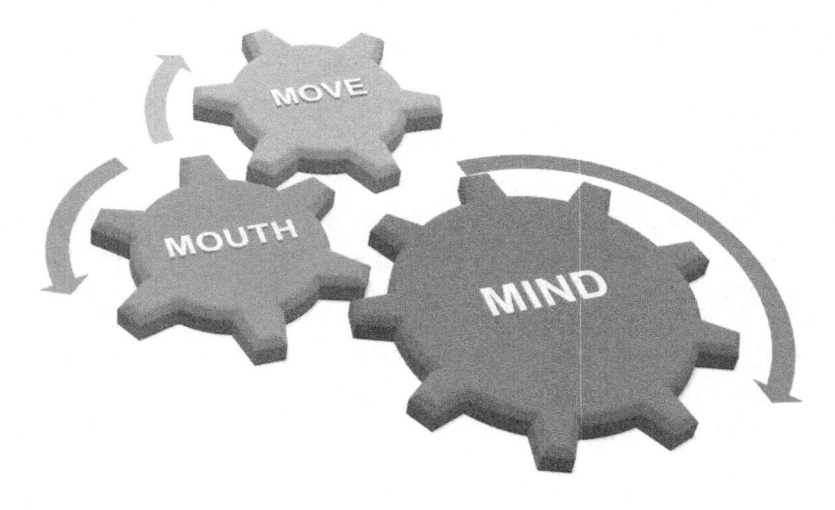

All three work closely together. If you continue to eat junk food and continue to live a sedentary life, it will affect your mind and sabotage the progress you desire.

Mind-Body Connection

There is a strong connection between the mind and the body. Neglect one, and the other will suffer. Your body responds negatively to emotions and eventually does not work the way it is supposed to when something is not right. People try to bury their heads in the sand while hiding their emotions from others and, most importantly, themselves. When a person is dealing with stress, it can lower their immune system response. The connection between stress and other illnesses suggests that stress can weaken the body's immune system. Stress can raise blood pressure temporarily; however, some studies show that stress can lead to long-term high blood pressure. Stress has always been a challenge for Tracy. She has learned to beat the adverse effects of stress, which includes exercising, reducing caffeine consumption, deep breathing exercises, avoiding process foods, prayer, and meditation. Since it is impossible to eliminate stress, practicing the techniques Tracy's discovered has reduced the impact of stress in her life and health.

Below are just a few health issues that can arise when the emotional and physical state is not in balance:

- High blood pressure
- Chest pain/shortness of breath
- Headaches
- Loss of appetite
- Being tired all the time
- Back pain or all-over aches and pain

- Constipation or diarrhea
- Insomnia or sleeping too much
- Heart irregularities
- Weight gain or loss

Any of these health issues will impact your longevity. Poor choices that you make daily could eventually cause the immune system to be weakened, increasing the risk of developing serious diseases. Proper balance of Mind, Mouth, and Move are required for optimum health no matter your current situation.

These strategies work! By accepting your current circumstances, along with changing your Mindset, you can add years to your life and find happiness that you only dreamed possible.

MIND - SMART MINDSET

Everyone has a different "WHY" —what is your "WHY"? Tracy believes the "mind" is the most important of the 3M Formula. When she found out she had diabetes, her "WHY" became crucial. She became determined not to allow this disease to kill her, and she would not suffer from the horrible complications that were guaranteed to happen.

What is your reason for getting healthy? Is it fear, afraid you will not see your grandkids grow up? What about wanting to travel after retirement, avoid being a burden to someone, or living a healthy, happy, fulfilled life? Whatever your reason, change your belief system now because this moment in time will never happen again. Thinking "It can't happen to me" or "I will take care of it tomorrow" will only cause disaster.

Putting your head in the sand or procrastinating could prevent you from changing your life right now and beginning the health journey you deserve.

Below are some of the strategies and techniques we have learned and implemented over the years:

Motivation

Find the real motive why you want to get healthy. Dig deep and find the actual reason. Once you determine your real motivation, visualize the "new" you. Can you see yourself living as a healthier person—the new real you? If your goal is to lose weight, imagine yourself at the ideal weight. If you want to start exercising, visualize yourself after six months of yoga, competing in a race, or playing in a tennis tournament, you have always wanted to do. Maybe your motivation is to eat healthy so you can increase your stamina. Picture yourself shopping on the perimeter of the grocery store (the healthiest section of the store). Visual imagery works wonders while it allows for "seeing" yourself in the future, precisely the way you want to be. Put pictures around your house or office for visual reminders of what you want. What works for us is having the mental image of the 86-year-old couple we met at the bottom of the Grand Canyon. They hike to the bottom twice a year and are a picture of health. That has been our motivating factor.

The Real Reason

Discovering the real reason why you want to make the change is critical. Is it because you genuinely want to make the change (internal motivation), or is another factor causing you to want the change (external motivation)? When understanding your right motivation for getting healthy, it allows you to understand the fact that you have a better chance of reaching your goals. If your doctor wants you to lose weight (external), you are less likely to stick with it. However, if the reason you want to make the change is that you want to enjoy life to the fullest (internal), then you are more likely to keep the goal and modify your life.

Reward System

Do not reward yourself with something to eat. Instead, find things you enjoy that you do not have time for, and when you reach the goal, indulge in this activity. For example, you want to start moving more. After two times of going to the gym, walking around the block, and lifting old milk jugs filled with water (a great way to save money on weights) for x number of days, treat yourself to 15 minutes of your favorite book or a magazine. Stop thinking of food (especially desserts) as a reward and look for alternatives. For example, enjoy a bubble bath, take a power nap, treat yourself to a massage, watch a movie, plan a night out with friends, or put a gold star by the goal you have accomplished.

Support

Positive support is critical when changing from an unhealthy life to one of health and power. Find a friend or a family member that will help you with accountability and will be a reinforcement when feeling tempted to fall back into old, bad habits. Everyone needs help occasionally, but especially during hard times. Having a strong group of people supporting you will help you to live longer and cope with life challenges, and you will not have to go through life alone. According to WebMD, a recent study[1] suggests that of 1,500 older people who participated in the study, those with a large group of friends lived longer than those without friends by a whopping 20%. When you have a strong, positive, healthy social support, you will have fewer heart problems and immune issues as well as lower levels of cortisol. Having friends also increases the sense of belonging, along with providing a purpose in one's life.

If you do not come up with your "WHY," you are more likely to stay on the couch and not exercise, eat the wrong food, and will not make the necessary changes to live a healthy life. Since your "WHY" is a motivating factor for success, if you do not know your "WHY," then make that your first goal.

We've all heard "you are what you eat," but we believe, "you think like you eat," too. When you fill your body with processed foods and not vegetables and fruit, it affects your mind. Several studies have found a correlation between a diet high in processed foods, fast foods, high fructose corn syrup, and sugars and weakened brain function along with the development of depression.

Coaching

There is value in getting the help of an expert who can coach and encourage you through the transformation. Professional athletes, along with other successful people, hire coaches to help them reach their goals. A good coach will listen, encourage, challenge, motivate, help you make better decisions, and guide you to the healthier life you desire.

www.LongevityCodes.com

Tracy has been coaching for many years and has seen remarkable changes in her clients. If you find yourself recently diagnosed, stuck, and not getting the results you desire, a health coach might be what you need to get you over the hump.

Finding the right coach can be a challenge. Be sure to talk with several coaches before making a choice. At the risk of sounding self-serving (since Tracy is a trained Wellness Coach, Certified Personal Trainer, and Lead Certified Longevity Health Coach), we feel having a coach who really understands is extremely valuable. Having dealt with diabetes (Type 1, the most challenging) for over 40 years successfully without complications, this puts her in an ideal position to guide those wanting to live a longer, healthier life. Consider her and her team if you need help and are at the point where you need a coach to help you reach your health goals:

Learn more about the Longevity Coaching Program at: www.LongevityCodes.com.

It starts with the Mind. Because it works closely together if you do not eat or move correctly, it will affect your Mind and sabotage the progress you desire.

Your immune system can be weakened by your poor emotional health and increase your risk of developing a serious illness.

This book is all about finding the proper balance of Mind, Mouth, and Move to help you have optimum health no matter your current diagnosis.

We have already shared how Tracy's mindset has helped her beat the odds. Take the next chapters seriously because finding the balance will add years to your life and life to your years.

MOUTH - SMART EATING

Smart eating is critical to having good health and a longer life. Diagnosed in the 1970s, with diabetes, Tracy learned the importance of eating only certain foods. She had not yet discovered the importance of "eat to live, not live to eat."

When choosing foods that help you and not hurt you, your energy levels increase. Also, your blood sugars remain level, and weight loss is often associated with this strategy. Tracy typically practices eating low glycemic foods. For a Free Report on the glycemic go to: www.TracyHerbert.com

The Right Choice

Maintaining and losing weight is based on burning more calories than the intake of calories. Consider the impact of metabolism since all calories are not equal. Diets providing less caloric intake along with incorporating an active lifestyle helps with the longevity. Glycemic Index should not be used alone in determining what to eat. Consider other nutritional factors such as total calories, portion size, amount of fats, fiber, vitamins, etc. Consult your physician or medical team when choosing a diet. For diabetics and pre-diabetics, low glycemic foods offer several benefits, including blood sugar management, weight reduction, and help in maintaining an active and healthy lifestyle.

When you eat the typical American breakfast a few hours later, your blood sugars spike, and several hours later, they fall, with or without diabetes. Because of eating this way, you feel sluggish. Replace those high carb breakfasts with salads, lean protein, and healthy fats! Learning these strategies has helped us transform our breakfast. We have more energy throughout the morning and are completely satisfied and remain full until midafternoon. What is the secret? We have a shake consisting of the following: unsweetened almond milk, cube approximately an inch of ginger root, chia seeds, hemp seeds, flax seeds, organic cocoa powder, organic protein powder, kale, spinach, peppermint oil, cinnamon oil, and ice. For several years Tracy has incorporated snacking on a green apple (remember, an apple a day keeps the doctor away) along with nuts, berries, and fresh vegetables daily. Her blood sugars remain level, and she feels energized. It has eliminated the sluggish feelings she used to experience before making the switch. It also reduces hunger pains and cravings, improves mental clarity, and achieves almost perfect blood glucose levels, which makes her the happiest.

The countries with the typical Western diet, consisting of processed and refined foods and sugars, proves to have more people with depression. Compared to those who eat the Mediterranean and standard Japanese meal plans consisting of more vegetables, fruits, fish, and seafood with only small amounts of lean meats and dairy products.

Ditch the soft drinks for tea! Drinking one cup of black or green tea daily can reduce the risk of heart disease. By making the switch, it can decrease the buildup of plaque commonly associated with cardiovascular disease versus those who do not drink any tea. Another benefit of drinking tea is that it can reduce your risk of certain types of cancer and can lower blood pressure and cholesterol. Not to mention making the switch to tea helps to avoid the dangers of high fructose corn syrup in regular soft drinks and the toxic chemicals found in artificial sweeteners. Of course, getting plenty of exercise and choosing healthy food options helps reduce heart disease and the others mentioned above.

Having a well-hydrated body is critical to a healthy life. If at first, you don't enjoy drinking water, add lemon, limes, or a slice of cucumber to give it an added zest. Drinking water also reduces hunger pains. When you feel hungry, most of the time, it is because you are dehydrated. Drinking a glass of water before a meal will help you differentiate between real hunger and dehydration. Another benefit of drinking a glass of water before a meal is that it will likely reduce the number of calories you consume. The body is composed of approximately 60% water. Each day you lose water by evaporation from the skin, urine, and breathing. Water is critical to bodily functions such as circulation, digestion, transporting nutrients, and maintaining body temperature. Muscles require adequate fluids to function correctly. For the kidneys to work perfectly, an appropriate amount of water is necessary. Water is also essential to prevent constipation. The current recommendations for water intake is half of your body weight in ounces.

Being Prepared

Preparation is the key to making healthy choices. It takes more time upfront, but by having healthy options available at home, at the office, and in the car, it makes it easier to stay on target. For example, we always have a water bottle with us everywhere we go and carry almonds, walnuts, and pecans for a healthy snack option. Always have a snack and drink plenty of water before going to the grocery store. By practicing this strategy, it will help you avoid impulse shopping. Each week we cut up various fresh vegetables and place them in sandwich bags, which helps speed up packing lunches and extra goodies to put in our salads.

Eating a small salad or something healthy before going to a party will give you the power before being tempted by unhealthy options that are abundant. Being successful at a party requires decisions before leaving the house. Simply predetermine what you will or will not eat or drink. To avoid being tempted, decide in advance to order a salad, protein, or other healthy options even if friends or family choose unhealthy options. This way, by planning before leaving the house, we have a goal and are prepared.

Plate Size – This is critical for good health!

The people who live the longest eat fewer calories. Fill at least one half of the plate with leafy greens and the other half with healthy fats, protein, and non-starchy carbohydrates. We enjoy broccoli, tomatoes, cauliflower, and other delicious foods that help us "eat to live, not live to eat!" On occasion, we will have a sweet potato, which is lower on the glycemic index and offers lots of healthy nutrients.

MOVE - SMART MOVEMENT

In this country, people just do not move enough! Sitting disease is the new smoking and is partially the cause of the

www.LongevityCodes.com

epidemic rise in Heart Disease, Type 2 diabetes, and obesity. Some researchers have found that sitting too much can be compared to the ill effects of smoking. By following these simple suggestions covered here, you will find strategies to help you move from a sedentary life to an active, healthy lifestyle. Having someone you enjoy doing things with will help keep you motivated. We like to change things up as not to get bored. Remember to start slow and let your body adapt. Starting too quickly can lead to injury and burnout. Always check with your doctor before starting or increasing an exercise program.

Following the strategies below will help jumpstart your road to getting healthy:

- To prevent sitting too long, set the alarm for every 50 minutes and get up, stretch, and walk around.
- Instead of sending an email, walk to their office to discuss the matter with a co-worker.
- In the office setting, consider having walking meetings.
- Get a stand-up desk.
- Stand while talking on the phone. Tracy likes to march in place while talking on the phone.
- Get up and move during TV commercials.
- Instead of meeting friends for lunch, take a walking lunch, and stop for a salad.
- Park farther away from the door. (Remember. it's not lucky to get a front-row parking spot; it's unhealthy.)
- Take the stairs instead of using elevators or escalators

www.LongevityCodes.com

Consult Your Healthcare Provider

For the effective management of your health and longevity, exercise is a must. Still, before starting any physical activity check with your doctor. Physicians will advise about your heart health and it is essential if you have developed narrowed arteries (atherosclerosis), cardiovascular problems, or hypertension (high blood pressure) to consult with your doctor.

Choose a Reasonable Exercise Plan

Set realistic goals, and gradually increase the quantity and intensity of exercise. Stay motivated and follow a healthy and practical exercise routine. You can also select easy and enjoyable activities like dancing, aerobics, cycling, tennis, swimming, walking, yoga, working in the yard, and anything that gets you up and moving. Finding an excellent personal trainer who can provide proper exercise strategies, techniques, and accountability will help push you to the next level of your health journey.

Keep Hydrated

Drink plenty of water throughout the day. Pay special attention and hydrate yourself before, during, and after exercise. Avoid working out in extremely hot or cold weather conditions.

Aerobic Exercises

Aerobic exercises are on top of the list of best activities for heart health. The National Institutes of Health[2] (NIH) has suggested approximately 150 minutes of aerobic exercise each week. Aerobic exercise increases insulin sensitivity in the body and helps to strengthen the heart, muscles, and bones. It also relieves stress, improves blood circulation, and reduces the risk for heart diseases by lowering blood sugar, cholesterol, and blood pressure.

The recommended length for a daily aerobic activity is roughly 30 minutes. You can do this time in one segment or break it down into 10-minute intervals. Aerobic activities include the following:

- Walking (mainly brisk walking)
- Cycling
- Jogging/Running
- Dancing
- Aerobics
- Stair climbing
- Hiking
- Tennis
- Basketball
- Swimming
- Gardening
- Yardwork and housework

Strength/Resistance Training

Once you have integrated aerobic exercise into your routine, do not forget strength training, which is critical as you age. Practice strength training at least two days a week in addition to aerobics. Strength or resistance training helps build stronger muscles and bones in addition to improving insulin sensitivity and lowering blood glucose. It also helps in preventing osteoporosis and bone fractures. Strength training should be practiced for roughly 20-30 minutes a day and two to three days a week.

Strength training activities include the following:

- Weightlifting or training
- Lifting free weights or using weight machines at a gym
- Home workouts such as pushups, sit-ups, planks, lunges, and squats, etc.

Balance Training

As you age, balance is critical. Without proper balance, it impacts your ability to stand, walk, and do the things you love. With the development of the complication of neuropathy, it gets difficult for people to maintain normal gait and balance, which is accompanied by loss of sensations, particularly in the feet. Balancing can help people in managing such problems. Achieving proper balance reduces falls and injuries and can be possibly eliminated.

Stretching and Flexibility Training

Flexibility training, such as stretching, can help in maintaining more flexible and stronger muscles and joints. When you become inflexible, it impacts your day to day activities. One of our "WHYs" for staying flexible is to get on the floor with our grandkids. Stretching before and after a workout can prevent muscle tears, aches, and soreness. Stretching exercises include basic or static stretches, dynamic stretching, moderate yoga, Pilates, Tai chi, etc.

Interval Training

Interval training is adding short periods of high-intensity activity into your regular exercise regimen. Interval training helps in improving stamina, effective control of blood sugar, and improving cardiovascular status. Interval training has been around for a long time, having been used mostly by athletes, until the past few years. Interval training improves lung function, reduces blood pressure faster than some aerobic type exercises. Recent studies have shown that older adults who are healthy but unfit were able to improve their blood glucose levels and insulin sensitivity after several weeks of interval training.

Fifteen to thirty seconds of high-intensity bursts of activity incorporated into regular training may help achieve the benefits of interval training. Tracy finds this type of exercise most beneficial with her busy schedule and for helping with her blood sugar control. Warm-up for five minutes, and then start to exercise as hard and fast as you can for 15-45 seconds. At this point, you should be out of breath and begin to slow back down but continue to move. Once your heart rate has fallen, complete another cycle. When starting, do only two or three high-intensity bursts, or as tolerated, and add additional cycles as you get stronger. Remember, cooling down is essential.

Be sure to check with your doctor before starting an exercise program. With interval training, you only want to do it once or twice a week unless an elite athlete. For beginners, just completing two or three interval series will provide a healthy workout option until building up to the full 15 minutes.

Longevity

There is a solid link between exercise and health, and regular exercise is associated with living a longer life. Even a moderate level of daily movement will help to lower your risk of death. Being physically active helps reduce the risk of obesity, cardiovascular disease, and diabetes and often reduces stress. Putting an exercise program in place is often difficult; however, do not use that as an excuse. If you think you don't have time, it's not convenient, or you don't enjoy it, change your thinking today. "Fitness is a journey, not a destination; you must continue for the rest of your life." Kenneth H. Cooper, MD, MPH

Following these steps will help you get on the right track:

- Find something you enjoy—because if you enjoy it, you will do it repeatedly.

- Do not overdo it when exercising. If you start too fast, you will suffer from burnout or injury. You will be more likely to stay with a fitness plan that involves more consistent workouts of moderate-intensity than one that is less frequent but more extreme.
    o Increase the length of time you work out slowly. Slow and steady wins the race, and developing an exercise plan is no exception.

- It's not too late to start.

www.LongevityCodes.com

- o According to the Center for Disease Control[3], only 20.8% of Americans participate in regular exercise, and that percentage decreases with age.
- o Consider the consequences of not beginning or increasing your exercise regime.

- Do you suffer from depression? For many people, an exercise prescription is just as valid as prescription medication (without any of the adverse side effects). But do not stop taking your medications without talking to your doctor first.

- Another benefit is that the mental decline slows down by eating healthy and exercising. Who doesn't want to grow old while staying mentally sharp?
  - o Weight-bearing exercise will help with bone loss. Did you know that after the age of 30, bone growth stops, and bone loss begins? Do not forget about the importance of Vitamin D. Brisk walking, running, lifting free weights, or resistant training on machines helps with bone loss.

- Exercise helps
  - o Improves balance (which is critical as you age), helps to control weight, boosts energy, improves mood, and helps with sleeping. Other benefits may include building self-esteem, ease arthritis, reduce stress, and helps to prevent, or control Type 2 diabetes. What most athletes enjoy is when they get the burst of endorphins, which is known as the "runner's high" and feel they can take on the world.

This 3M Formula works! No membership is necessary, and your doctor will be thrilled. Start slow and work on one area

www.LongevityCodes.com

before adding something else. You can do this! Start today and begin to see improvement in energy, sleep, and better health.

If you need help with any of these strategies or need a personal Longevity Codes Coach to help you with the process, go to: www.LongevityCodes.com

> Get additional FREE RESOURCES at
> # www.LongevityCodes.com

Chapter 7

Finding the Perfect Diet

Always consult your physician or other health care professional before changing your meal plan to determine if it is right for your needs. If you have a history of diabetes or take certain medications, this is particularly true. Do not change your meal plan if your physician or health care provider advises against it.

What is the perfect diet? Coaching clients ask Tracy this question all the time. With a new fad diet appearing weekly, it's understandable why this subject is so confusing.

One of the first steps towards longevity is to achieve a healthy body weight and stay there.

In a study of 500,000 healthy nonsmokers ages 50 to 70, a direct correlation was found between those who were overweight and those who died an early death. It's a simple formula, get to your ideal body weight, maintain it, practice healthy strategies, and you'll live longer.

A study[1] on morbidity and mortality identified 13 areas where obesity impacts life expectancy. Cancer and cardiovascular accounted the greatest risks from obesity.

Two-thirds of Americans are either overweight or obese. Typically, people gain weight over a long time, doesn't it make sense that they need to lose it over a long period? Those who are smart about losing weight the healthy way tend to keep it off longer.

www.LongevityCodes.com

The word diet is negative. The first three letters spell D-I-E. If you're overweight, getting to a healthy weight is a critical strategy for longevity. For living longer, consider replacing the word diet with a healthy eating plan. It's not a diet but a lifestyle!

Recognizing that no one is perfect, is paramount, and beating yourself up does not help. One day it's one step forward, and the next day it's two steps backward. Understanding that this is normal and how you respond makes all the difference. Forgive yourself and keep moving towards the health goals you desire.

When we use the term diet, we're not talking about some sort of quick fix eating program! Instead, it's foods consumed daily. Finding a quick and easy weight loss strategy is not recommended. What experts endorse is to establish a healthy lifestyle that helps you reach your longevity goals.

What is a proper healthy diet, especially for someone who's looking towards living a longer and healthier life?

Your daily food choices should include all these elements:

- Eat foods that help you and do not harm you while achieving a healthy body weight. It's essential to maintain an ideal body weight once reached. A large percentage of people who lose weight gain it back within six months and then some.
- Choose foods that support health at a cellular level. It includes foods that feed and promote healthy cells while avoiding and eliminating foods that cause cellular damage.
- Foods must help reduce inflammation. Excessive inflammation causes serious health issues, along with joint pain.

- Enjoy the right foods for success. When you find healthy foods you enjoy, eating them will make it easier to be a lifelong choice. Once reaching the ideal body weight, it's essential to keep these foods in your daily plan. When eating clean, you won't want to go back to the unhealthy choices because of the way it makes you feel.
- Choose the eating plan that helps avoid chronic health issues like heart disease, diabetes, cancer, arthritis, Alzheimer's, etc. Unhealthy eating and lifestyle choices often lead to many of these diseases. Preventing these lifestyle-related diseases helps you live longer.
- Pick foods low in heavy metals and toxins. It is impossible to eliminate every contamination but try to avoid exposure as much as possible. Organic foods are the best choice. When choosing fish, select wild-caught fish, which is known to be low in mercury.
- Find a diet that's unique for you and one you will enjoy. Our bodies are all different, and what works for one may not work for another. Don't select a diet based on the latest fad, but make sure it has scientific backing and that it works for you. There is no magic formula! You have a unique DNA and body chemistry that causes you to react to food differently than anyone else, test what works for you.

The Un-Diet

Eating less is a strategy we call the Un-Diet because it's not a diet or a meal plan; it's merely an approach to stop eating when you feel about 80% full. Longevity studies started as early as the 1930s when scientists began researching and studying mice and found they could live dramatically longer when they reduced the amount of food consumed.

Americans are obsessed with oversized portions, and this unhealthy approach is quickly spreading around the world. An average adult meal 30 years ago would be laughed at today and considered a kid's meal. Customers return to restaurants that serve excessive portion sizes by coming back for more. Everyone wants a good value when eating out, but we've gone to the extreme. Learning how to be satisfied with less, and stop eating before becoming full, helps us develop smart eating habits for longevity.

Now that you know it's vital for longer life to consume fewer calories, here are some popular diets to consider:

The Mediterranean Diet

Physicians around the world recommend this diet because it promotes longevity. People in the Mediterranean region live longer and have fewer health issues than those living in the United States. Their regime has a healthier balance of omega-3 (the good fats), with fresh fruits, veggies, whole grains, fish, olive oil, garlic, and drinking wine in moderation. This diet has less omega-6 oils (which is terrible if you consume too much or are out of balance), meat, and snack foods. People in this region are less likely to develop heart disease, diabetes, and other diet-related diseases. The Mediterranean diet might be the right place for you to start.

Atkins Diet

In 1972 Dr. Robert Atkins published his first book, and his diet is considered a Low Carb diet. What this program taught us is a high-fat low carb diet helps people lose weight, and is a useful tool for lowering cholesterol and triglycerides. This approach was revolutionary but contrary to the fat myth of the time. While this diet proved, you can lose weight and even improve cholesterol and triglycerides this diet should not be a long-term eating plan. Restricted intake of carbohydrates can be damaging over a long period; therefore, this would not be a diet for longevity. This plan, like all others, evolves, and their updates have made improvements.

The Ketogenic Diet

This diet uses fats rather than carbohydrates. The energy source for this diet consists of fats, a sufficient amount of protein, and low carbs. Originally designed to treat severe cases of epilepsy in children and is also now used by many people with diabetes to control blood sugars. Often called the Keto diet and is like the Atkins Diet and other low carb diets. Some experts are concerned there might be long-term health issues with consuming fewer healthy carbohydrates.

The Low Glycemic diet

The glycemic index is a measure of how foods spike your blood sugar. When your blood sugars spike quickly, your pancreas must produce even more insulin than usual. Think about the last time you ate a pizza or donut, and a few hours later, felt lethargic and wanted to take a nap. When this happens, your blood sugar spikes, insulin is released, and then you crash because of the overcompensation. The battle of eating this way can increase insulin resistance, which often leads to Type 2 diabetes. Want to lose weight? Want more energy? Choosing low glycemic foods is what Tracy recommends to all of her personal training clients and coaching clients. There's no way to go wrong when opting for low glycemic foods over high glycemic foods. Talk with your doctor because they will be 100% in favor of this diet strategy. Want more information on a low glycemic diet? For free resources, go to:

www.LongevityCodes.com

Using this strategy will change your life!

Paleo Diet

Using this approach takes you back to what your Hunter-Gatherer ancestors would have eaten. Eat anything that can be hunted or gathered like meats, fish, nuts, berries, seeds, and veggies. You can't go wrong using this approach because eliminating processed foods is suitable for living a longer, healthier life.

Blood Type Diet

Eating healthy foods for your blood type is the idea. Tracy found this to work well for her. Dr. Peter J. D'Amamo lays out guidelines of what you should eat in his book "Eat Right for Your Type." Of course, there are critics to using this approach, but it might be something to consider.

Vegan and Vegetarian

A lifestyle diet that helps people lose weight, and there is evidence it could be a good longevity strategy. Studies have shown that some people who live the longest, on average, eat very little meat, if any.

If you need help losing weight or are confused by all the different diet plans, go to the Longevity Codes website for free resources. The strategies offered at Longevity Codes doesn't require purchasing packaged meals or make you count points. Most plans require you to fit in a cookie-cutter approach. The Longevity Codes method is just the opposite. The big chain companies will help you lose weight, but their plans aren't sustainable over time. They don't teach lifestyle strategies without being on their program. Their mission is not like ours, where we want to work ourselves out of a job because you are successful and can do it on your own.

The diet plans we've covered all have pros and cons, and one type doesn't work for everyone. You're different, and you must find what works best for you and adjust to your unique circumstances.

Have you considered keeping a food journal to see what helps your body and what hurts your body? If you continue to eat foods that cause a mild or severe allergic reaction, it causes inflammation and other health issues. By keeping a food journal for two weeks and writing everything down, you'll be shocked at what you discover. Certain foods triggered Fred's digestive system, and he didn't realize it until keeping the journal. Write everything that goes into your mouth, including liquids. What many people discover is they don't drink near the amount of water they think they do. Water is essential to good health, and many times when you feel hungry, you are dehydrated. If you feel hungry, drink a glass of water and wait 15 minutes. Most of the time, the hunger pain goes away, and you were merely dehydrated.

Here's fundamental tools and strategies to help you find YOUR perfect longevity diet:

Start with low glycemic foods!

Choose foods high in good healthy fats, high in omega-3 fatty acids, and low in the bad guys like saturated fats, trans fats, hydronated oils, and stay away from processed foods.

A standard recommendation by nutritionists is to stay away from these five unhealthy white foods:

1. White bread
2. White potatoes
3. Table salt (but not all salt is bad use pink Himalayan sea salt that's full of healthy minerals)
4. White sugar
5. White rice

Stay away from processed foods as much as possible.

How do you find the perfect diet for you? Just what you're doing: you learn, you read, listen to podcasts, talk to a nutritionist, and speak with your doctor. You must take control of your health! Find the plan that works best for you.

> ***"The only way to keep your health is to eat what you don't want, drink what you don't like, and do what you'd rather not."***
> Mark Twain

www.LongevityCodes.com

That's funny and is true to start. Still, when you focus on your **why** for living a longer and healthier life, you learn to enjoy **eating, drinking, and doing** what works for your health and longevity goals.

You might have started reading this chapter, hoping to find your "magic pill" and discover the perfect diet. Sorry to disappoint you, but what we've done is provide you tools to help you identify your ideal **PERFECT LONGEVITY DIET**.

Check out
LONGEVITY CODES COACHING PROGRAM
www.LongevityCodes.com
Our **Longevity Codes Certified Coach** will help you implement the principles in this book and provide the tools and accountability you need to achieve fast results.

www.LongevityCodes.com

Chapter 8

Critical Cell Signaling

Imagine your house is on fire and you call the fire department. The fire station has everything needed to fight the blaze: the fire truck, firefighters, fire hose, and they have the skills necessary to put out the fire. Because of a weak phone signal, they cannot get the message needed to protect your house, and your home goes up in flames!

Like the fire analogy the focus is on the fire truck, not the communication system; similarly, the health and wellness industry fail when the focus is in the wrong place. Vitamins, minerals, antioxidants, and other supplements are examples of the tool but not the message reaching the cell. Of course, these are all necessary for optimal health, but they do not address the communication problem. When the body has the crucial cell signaling resources needed, it allows the cells to function correctly. What is this powerful resource? Redox Signaling Molecules!

Scientists have been trying to discover for years how the human cell works, what causes them to become damaged, diseased, and how you age. Three scientists won the Nobel Prize in 1998 for their discovery of Redox Signaling Molecules. They learned how redox signaling activates the antioxidants to signal genes in cells to combat cellular stress, fight off bacteria, and viruses. Most diseases are caused by cellular stress or oxidative stress in some way.

An oxidative stress study[1] showed reactive oxygen species (ROS) could cause a wide range of disorders that include

www.LongevityCodes.com

Alzheimer's, Parkinson's, aging, and other neural disorders. Free radical toxicity contributes to harming DNA, inflammation, and tissue damage.

Because the body has 75 trillion cells, it is essential to lower oxidative stress to remain healthy. Any breakdown in this complex communication network between your cells prevents good health!

Redox Signaling Molecules are native to the body and made from the saltwater found inside your cells. The problem is that after reaching puberty, you lose about 10% of your capacity to make these critical molecules every decade. At our age, we are making about half what it did when we were kids, which explains why we don't recover from illness or physical activity like we used to.

Now the great news! There's a way to supplement and increase the much-needed supply of these essential molecules.

Is this science for real? Being the skeptic that Tracy is, along with her lifelong pursuit of health and wellness, she quickly started researching. After discovering thousands of peer-reviewed articles and scientific studies on Redox Signaling Molecules, it convinced us the science is real. After all, the Nobel Prize is not awarded to just anyone.

Once thought to be a byproduct of mitochondria energy production, redox molecules turned out to have a more significant impact on cellular health. Scientists now know that it is a critical part of the cell communication system and vital in every function of cellular health.

Healthy cell signaling throughout the body is foundational to cellular rejuvenation and renewal. At the time of this

www.LongevityCodes.com

writing, there are over 15,000 peer-reviewed articles, 1,200 books explaining how Redox Signaling Molecules are involved in virtually every central body system, and over 18,000 cited publications in PubMed.

Human genes have the blueprints and instructions for cellular health throughout the body! But living in a world full of environmental toxins which stresses our genes and turns them off with catastrophic results. These stats are for the United States, but is also a global problem:

- 50 Million Americans suffer from autoimmune challenges from more than 100 autoimmune diseases.[2]
- Fifty-four million or 23% have arthritis which is an inflammatory condition.[3]
- Heart disease is the leading cause of death, and 647,000 Americans (1 in 4 deaths) die from it each year.[4]
- 61% have weekly GI symptoms, including heartburn/reflux, abdominal pain, bloating, diarrhea, constipation, and others.[5]

Is it possible to supplement and get more Redox Signaling Molecules? Yes!

The challenge was that Redox Signaling Molecules were highly reactive and fleeting. For a long-time, science had declared it was impossible to stabilize these molecules outside of the body. It took almost two decades, and tens of millions of dollars for research before a group of scientists led by an atomic Medical Physicist achieved "the impossible." For the first time, scientists created and stabilized the powerful Redox Signaling Molecules outside of the body.

www.LongevityCodes.com

They started with only salt and water, just like what's inside every human cell, and passed it through a complex, heavily patented three-day process. The saltwater is broken down and restructured into trillions of Redox Signaling Molecules. This process of stabilization launched a company that has exclusive Redox Signaling Technology, which means there is no competition.

Redox Signaling Molecule supplement is not a treatment or cure for any disease or medical condition. However, in an eight-week study, this supplement was shown to activate five critical gene signaling pathways by up to 31%, which in turn can positively impact these five major areas:

- Improve immune system health
- Help maintain a healthy inflammatory response
- Help maintain cardiovascular health and support arterial elasticity
- Improve digestive health
- Modulate hormone balance

And this is only scratching the surface. For example, just one of these genes tested can influence 15 additional pathways, including those involving insulin signaling, thyroid hormones, and spinal cord injuries. Although there are no antioxidants in this product with Redox Signaling Molecules, its impact on antioxidant health is significant!

World Class Athletes using Redox Signaling Molecule supplementation reported going further, faster, and longer. While using this product they experienced improvements in endurance, strength, recovery, and mental focus. A university study with mice found those who drank Redox Signaling Molecules for only seven days found their stamina increased by 29%.

www.LongevityCodes.com

Redox Signaling Molecules has made a big difference for Fred. It takes longer to reach his maximum heart rate during interval training and recovers faster. His once extreme joint pain is now gone, he sleeps better, and his mood is better. Tracy found that her sleep is like it was when she was a teenager.

As mentioned earlier, the company that figured out how to stabilize these molecules and put them in a liquid you can drink or apply has a complicated patented process.

After millions of dollars spent on research and studies on this technology, it has proven to be 100% safe with zero levels of toxicity. There is no other source for Redox Signaling Molecule supplementation.

Want to learn more about Redox Signaling Molecules? Go to: www.LongevityCodes.com/redox

Gary Samuelson, Ph.D., an Atomic Medical Physicist, discovered how to stabilize redox signaling molecules into a form to supplement. He said: "This technology has the potential to spearhead the greatest advances in health we have ever seen."

"*Our physical health is dependent on our cellular health!*"
Fred Herbert

Redox Signaling Molecule supplementation is our top Longevity Code Strategy, for improved cellular health and anti-aging.

Chapter 9

Reversing Biological Age

Did you realize at the age of 50, you could have the biological age of a 70-year-old? And the opposite is true. You could be 50 and have the biological age of a 30-year-old.

Tao Porchon-Lynch began practicing yoga in 1926 at the age of eight and retired teaching at the age of 96. Imagine her biological age?

Chronological age is how long you have been alive, but what's frightening could be your biological age?

The health of your cells and organs determine biological age.

Want to stop or reverse the biological age? These strategies are guaranteed to help:

Mitochondria

The mitochondria are the little power plants in the cells that produce energy Adenosine triphosphate or (ATP). Energy from the mitochondria keeps everything working; when ATP stops, the body dies. Every cell has mitochondria, and some have hundreds, while others have thousands. Mitochondria production slows down as you age, impacting your brain, heart, muscle mass, and your energy level.

Proven strategies on how to boost the mitochondria:

- High-intensity exercise

- Ketogenic diet
- Cell boosting supplements
- Intermittent fasting
- Healthy fats
- Anti-inflammatory diet

For more information on mitochondria see Chapter 14.

Increase Autophagy

Autophagy means self-devouring. It is the process of breaking down unhealthy and damaged cells to repair and rebuild healthy ones.

Two strategies to boost autophagy are High-Intensity Interval Training and Intermittent Fasting. These should be at the top of your action list if you are not currently doing them.

Chapter 18 has additional ways to improve autophagy.

Manage Stress

Regions around the world, whose citizens live the longest, have lower stress levels compared to those living in high-stress environments.

Adverse impact of stress includes:

- Heart disease
- High blood pressure
- Weakened immune system
- Autoimmune diseases
- Diabetes

- Obesity
- Gastrointestinal disorders
- Skin irritation
- Respiratory infections
- Insomnia
- Burnout
- Depression
- Anxiety disorders

It's no wonder stress plays a significant role in the biological age. Stress is handled differently by everyone. How do you handle stress? Do you hold it in or explode?

How to effectively deal with stress:

- Exercise
- Meditation
- Improve sleep
- Yoga
- Take a walk in the park or woods
- Talking to someone. Friends, family, or a counselor
- Eat a healthy diet
- Reduce caffeine
- Have fun and do things that make you laugh
- Hot bath or sauna
- Deep breathing exercise
- Soothing music
- Pet your dog
- Keep a gratitude journal

Find strategies to help lower your stress and practice them regularly.

Improve Cell Signaling

Another biological age reversal strategy is replenishing the Redox Signaling Molecules in your body. Your ability to produce these critical signaling molecules decline about 10% per decade. Boosting Redox Signaling Molecules improve gene expressions in five ways:

- Improved immune system
- Healthy hormone modulation
- A better inflammatory response
- Better digestive function
- And it helps the cardiovascular system

Learn more about this Nobel Prize-winning technology in Chapter 8.

Longevity Diet

As Tracy always says, "Eat to live don't live to eat!" Mimic the diets of those who live the longest. Studies of centenarians show commonalities in their diets which include:

- Mostly a plant-based diet
- Low in meat proteins and some cases no meat at all
- Healthy fats like olive oil
- Limit sugar and processed foods only to special occasions
- High in whole grains and beans
- Healthy berries like blueberries
- And includes healthy raw unsalted nuts like almonds, pistachios, and walnuts

Review Chapter 7 to find your "Finding the Perfect Diet."

Maintain an Ideal Body Weight

That is easier said than done. Obesity is a negative factor in cellular aging because it makes systems work harder to keep up. The extra burden on essential organs causes people to age prematurely.

According to a study by the National Institutes of Heath[1], obesity can shorten lifespan by up to 14 years. Deaths linked to obesity include heart disease, cancer, and diabetes. This epidemic is serious because two-thirds of Americans are overweight or obese.

This prescription is simple! Get to and maintain an ideal body weight. If this is an issue for you, consider this a priority. Practicing this strategy will help to turn back your biological clock, which allows you to live a longer, healthier, and a more active life.

Get Quality Sleep

Sleep is critical for good health and longevity.

A study[2] showed a correlation between not having enough quality sleep and a reduced lifespan.

For more information on improving sleep see Chapter 21.

3M Formula

To improve our biological age, we practice Tracy's 3M Formula. Mind, Mouth, and Move. Everything we have covered for improving our biological age fits into one of these three categories. The 3M Formula is closely intertwined and impossible to do one without the other. For example, not having the right mindset prevents people from exercising and eating healthy. When eating poorly, others often forgo choosing the healthiest food options and become less motivated to exercise. If you do not exercise, it negatively affects mood and food choices. It's cyclical and goes hand in hand.

Action items to have a biological age younger than your chronological age:

- Take care of your mitochondria
- Promote autophagy
- Manage your stress
- Improve cell signaling with redox signaling molecules
- Eat a diet like the centenarians do
- Get to and maintain your ideal body weight
- Get good quality sleep
- Follow Tracy's 3M Formula Mind Mouth and Move

Chapter 10

Beat Stress for Better Health

Not all stress is harmful, but chronic stress impacts health and aging negatively.

Tracy found this to be true the hard way. Ten years ago, she was working a high-stress job in corporate America and developed a strange heartbeat. Her doctor for over 30 years could not figure out what was wrong and immediately called a cardiologist. What scared Tracy, even more, was the fearful look in his eyes. She had an appointment the next morning, and the doctor instructed: "don't work out or watch anything stressful."

The cardiologist ran every test in the book. While doing the nuclear stress test, the doctor was shocked and asked another cardiologist to come in and watch. Tracy felt tremendous and could not figure out what was wrong. After the test, he said, "your heartbeat straightened out while exercising," and about 15 minutes later, it returned to the crazy heartbeat again. Tracy thought the nuclear stress test was fun (she has a different idea of fun than most people) because they kept increasing the treadmill speed and elevation, allowing her to feel great with no heart issues.

Tracy's cardiac catheterization came back clear. However, the cardiologist said, "your heart is fine, but if you don't take control of your stress, it's going to kill you!" Hearing this is when she first understood the importance of reducing stress and has been researching and practicing the principles shared in this chapter.

www.LongevityCodes.com

Chronic stress linked to:

- Heart disease
- Diabetes
- Depression
- Obesity
- Accelerated aging
- Premature death
- Alzheimer's disease

According to the National Institute of Mental Health[1], chronic stress can disrupt the immune system, digestion, sleep, and cardiovascular system.

A report from the Department of Psychiatry at the University of California[2] reported that while stress has a protective function if overwhelmed, it causes damage such as oxidative stress and shortening of telomere length. Shorter telomere length is associated with a shorter lifespan.

Chronic stress negatively impacts your body, mood, and behavior.

Body:

- Headaches
- Muscle tension or pain
- Chest pain
- Fatigue
- Stomach upset
- Sleep problems

Mood:

- Anxiety
- Lack of motivation or focus

- Feeling overwhelmed
- Irritability or anger
- Sadness or depression

Behavior:

- Overeating or undereating
- Restlessness
- Angry outbursts
- Misuse of drugs or alcohol
- Tobacco use
- Social withdrawal
- Exercising less often

Chronic psychological stress is linked[3] to accelerated aging, an increase of disease, and premature death.

The picture might seem bleak, but there are things you can do to reduce chronic stress. These tools have worked wonders for Tracy and her coaching clients.

Practice Breathing

It might sound funny, but there is a right way to breathe. Most of us take shallow breaths and do not fully utilize the oxygen capacity of our lungs. To learn how to breathe correctly, sit up straight, and close your eyes. Place your hand on the belly to make sure you are getting a deep abdominal breath. Inhale through the nose and then exhale through the mouth. Tracy practices visualization during this process and imagines pure, clean air entering through the nose and filling her lungs. While exhaling, she pictures viruses, toxins, stress, and other unhealthy things leaving her body.

Deep breathing also helps to lower heart rate and blood pressure.

Exercise

One of our favorite ways to reduce stress is exercise. Believe it or not, exercise can be relaxing but only if it is something you enjoy. For example, some may prefer gardening or walking, while others enjoy bicycling or running. When you find activities you enjoy, you will continue to do it.

How does exercise reduce stress?

It reduces your body's stress hormones like cortisol and adrenaline. Many athletes' favorite part of exercising is achieving the "runner's high," with the endorphins lifting their moods, helping them feel invincible while reducing stress. When the kids were teenagers and saw Tracy exhibiting signs of stress, they would say, "mom go run!" They were not disrespectful but knew how exercise helped their mom reduce stress.

Stay Connected

Another way to reduce stress is by staying connected with family or friends. Find ways to engage with people who are positive, encouraging, and understanding. Make it a priority to reach out to people and stay connected; it's good for your health. Together we're stronger, and we don't want anyone to be sad, alone, or without hope. The people who live the longest have solid social connections.

Music

Another thing to lower stress is listening to upbeat music. Experiment and find music that calms and brings peace. Next time you start feeling anxious, turn on the music.

Laugh

"Laughter is the best medicine!" Laughing helps you stay positive and lowers stress levels. Try to watch something funny before going to bed to end the day on a positive note. Some people have even cured diseases through laughter. Give it a try for longevity!

Other issues resulting from chronic stress are skin problems, digestive issues, and autoimmune disorders. When living with chronic stress, your adrenal glands become overworked, which causes all types of complications. Do not wait until stress negatively impacts your health before acting. Make it a priority to get stress under control if it is an issue for you. Your health is at stake!

Get additional FREE RESOURCES at
www.LongevityCodes.com

Chapter 11

Build a Strong Immune System

Longevity requires a robust immune system that can fight off every invader that tries to attack.

What protects you from cancer cells and other deadly invaders?

Your immune system!

The immune system is what protects you from the bad guys. Invaders such as toxins, bacteria, viruses, and fungi create a network of poor health. The immune system has two parts: The innate system you are born with, and the acquired immune system you build over time. When functioning correctly, your immune system produces cells called antibodies to protect you from specific invaders. Once exposed to an invader, your immune system goes to work to recognize the threat and defend against it. How immunizations work is to train the body to build the necessary antibodies to fight off the invasion.

The immune system is like a Superhero! Each time your body's immune system fights off an infection, it becomes more robust and able to fight off similar threats the next time. The first time a person sees a sign of infection, they immediately panic and think, "I need to start taking antibiotics." When this happens, it does not allow the immune system time to build up strength.

It is helpful to have a basic understanding of how the immune system works; in this book, we will not get too technical. That's just it; it's a complicated and underappreciated system that works behind the scenes. Multiple organs produce the cells in your immune system, such as:

- Tonsils
- Bone marrow
- Adenoids
- Lymph nodes
- Lymphatic vessels
- Spleen
- Thymus

Why is this important to longevity!

As you age, your immune system is reduced and makes you more vulnerable to infections and disease. The mechanisms that cause this are not clear, but some scientists see a correlation with the decrease of T cell production. As the thymus ages and atrophies, it produces fewer T cells that fight off infections.

While it is true the average person has a weakened immune response as they age, we believe we can all be the exception to this rule. But you must be ready to act! Because of practicing the strategies found in this book, Fred has a stronger immune system in his mid-sixties, then when he was younger. It is the same thing for Tracy. Writing this book became a passion of ours to share everything we have learned by researching and practicing these strategies. By reading this book, you join us on a mission to live a longer and healthier life.

The pursuit of building a healthy immune system starts now. This way, you can avoid respiratory issues, heart disease, mental decline, and all the other issues typically associated with aging.

Do you want a healthy immune system?

The answer to accomplish this question comes in two forms:

- Avoid and stay away from things that hurt the immune system
- Cling to and practice things that support it

First, things to avoid that can weaken or damage the immune system.

Top of the list, STRESS!

Modern medicine has finally recognized the Mind/Body connection. The whole study of the placebo effect proves the mind can help with the healing process. It is also well documented that negative mindset, grief, anger, and chronic stress can make a person sick and unhealthy.

Studies show[1] that as we age, our bodies have trouble mounting the immune responses needed to react to stressors. Psychological stressors can cause you to have accelerated aging beyond your chronological age. Aging researchers have linked shortened telomere length with chronic stress and increased disease.

Chronic stress is a killer; it's terrible for your health and can negatively affect your immune system too. If stress is an issue for you, research and find ways to get it under control. Meditation and deep breathing exercises help Tracy ease the stress that wreaks havoc in her life if she does not control it.

Smoking

Smoking kills and lowers the defense system. If you smoke stop! Your future self will thank you for it.

Alcohol

If you drink, drink in moderation.

Stay away from sugar

When consuming too much sugar, it impacts your immune system and the cells needed to attack bacteria and infections. Sugar has many adverse effects on your body, eat it sparingly and only on special occasions and not as the norm.

Avoiding Germs

Limiting exposure to germs can help reduce the risk of getting sick. The best way to take control and keep bacteria away is by frequently washing hands, using disinfectants, and avoid touching the face. Another area often overlooked is to bypass foods not appropriately prepared. Salmonella is something you do not want!

Things that Improve the Immune System:

First up! Nutrition – A healthy immune system starts with giving your body the necessary building blocks for an excellent cellular health foundation. These foods help to improve your immune system and are best for overall good health:

- Broccoli and other cruciferous vegetables should be a staple in daily meal preparation, packed with vitamins, fiber, and antioxidants.
- Red bell peppers have double the Vitamin C of citrus and a great source of beta carotene.
- Garlic has strong immune-boosting qualities that many believe comes from the concentration of heavy sulfur-containing compounds.
- Spinach packed with antioxidants and beta carotene should be a staple in your kitchen. We eat spinach most mornings in our greens and protein shake.
- Ginger is excellent for decreasing inflammation and can help reduce chronic pain.
- Green tea is a potent antioxidant and excellent source of L-theanine amino acids that aid in producing T cells that fight germs.
- Sunflower seeds are incredibly high in Vitamin E that helps to regulate and maintain your immune system.
- The list goes on and on, but others to keep in mind are:
    - Turmeric
    - Kiwi
    - Papaya
    - Almonds
    - Poultry
    - Shellfish

All of these have nutritional properties that help the immune system.

Redox Signaling Molecules

Discussed in Chapter 8, another vital strategy for improving your cellular health is adding Redox Signaling Molecules. To learn more about Redox Signaling Molecules, check out www.LongevityCodes.com/redox

Autophagy

The no-cost plan to trigger autophagy is FASTING. Intermittent fasting is a tool in our health toolbox to promote autophagy, which in turn destroys our weak and damaged cells. Give it a try! For more information on Autophagy see Chapter 18.

Sleep

Sleep is a powerhouse for good health, longevity, and helps to build a more robust immune system. Researchers[2] using epidemiology studies have found a correlation between lack of sleep and increased risk of infectious disease, which is associated with a lowered immune system.

Having the right view of sleep and relaxation is significant. Neither is a waste of time, nor should these be thought of negatively. During sleep, your body can rejuvenate and build a powerful immune system. The importance of sleep is covered in Chapter 21.

Exercise

If exercise is a dirty word for you, get over it because it's an essential strategy for improving overall health while building a more reliable immune system.

Within the immune system, there's a sweet spot between being a couch potato and a marathon runner[3]. Overtraining or too little exercise can weaken your immune system. Living a long, healthier life is imperative, and movement increases longevity. There are lots of health benefits of living an active life and including exercise as part of your health strategy is critical. It will help to improve the immune system. Chapter 19 covers fitness in greater detail.

Gut Health

Researchers[4] have found a correlation between gut health and the immune system. Having a healthy gut microbiota and a powerful, healthy immune system go hand in hand.

Fred started taking probiotics 20 years ago to improve his gut health and to provide the beneficial bacteria he needed. He used to be sick all the time with multiple sinus infections, along with the flu. Now, he rarely gets sick. Tracy started seeing similar results when she started taking probiotics 18 years ago. Wow, what an improvement in both of our lives. For more information on improving gut health see Chapter 15.

The Verdict

The evidence for getting serious about your immune system is compelling. A healthy immune system is a crucial element

www.LongevityCodes.com

for living a longer and healthier life. Do not take good health for granted! Start today to begin to incorporate some or all the strategies in this chapter.

Want to build a healthy immune system? Start by reviewing your nutrition, quality of sleep, exercise routine, and work on your healthy gut. Be sure to limit exposure to unhealthy toxins; they are everywhere. Stay away from eating too much sugar, stop smoking, limit the amount of alcohol consumed, and reduce stress to improve the immune system.

No doubt, a robust, healthy immune system will help your efforts toward longevity.

Check out
LONGEVITY CODES COACHING PROGRAM
www.LongevityCodes.com
Our **Longevity Codes Certified Coach** will help you implement the principles in this book and provide the tools and accountability you need to achieve fast results.

Chapter 12

Eliminate Aches and Pains

What's that the number one complaint expressed by people as they age?

Typically, it's something like "oh my aching back, knees, hips," and the list goes on and on? You name it, and many older people share their complaints with anyone willing to listen.

But does it have to be that way?

Could you be the exception?

Being in pain all the time is not something you want and is a common fear with aging.

It doesn't have to be that way. Living an active and pain-free life is achievable, and using these tools may help you as it has us.

Does this describe you? Are you starting to feel some of the aches and pains of aging? Many people needing back, knee, or hip replacement surgery have poor outcomes. Could a negative mindset be a factor in the outcome? An arthroscopic knee surgery study[1] compared a placebo procedure against an actual meniscus tear repair. The result showed those receiving the conventional surgery compared to those who had the "fake" operation fared no better.

Great news! Whether you are already suffering from age-related pains or you want to prevent it from happening, the remedies are all the same.

The following strategies help to eliminate aches and pains:

Ideal Body Weight

Could you be a victim of gravity? That's right, and it's all gravity's' fault. If you lived in a zero-gravity environment, those extra pounds would not take such a toll on your joints. For every ten extra pounds of body weight you carry, it puts an additional 30 pounds of pressure on your knee joints. In the United States, two-thirds of the citizens are either overweight or obese. People are doing it to themselves! An Orthopedic Surgeon we know frequently tells his patients when overweight to lose some weight before considering surgery. He recommends being patient, lose some weight, and see if the pain subsides. This surgeon loses lots of surgery patients but has the patient's best interest at heart. Although this might not be the quick fix many are looking for but losing a few pounds will pay off and may eliminate the need for surgery.

That's our prescription, too – get to your ideal body weight. Eat fewer calories and exercise to become lean has been associated with longevity in countless studies.

Step one – get to a perfect weight!

Flexibility!

The older we get, the more important it is to realize that if there is a fountain of youth, flexibility is it. As people age, it's common to see older people hunched over, use a walker, taking mini-steps, and have difficulties getting in the car. Do something every day to keep joints flexible to avoid this happening to you. Make a deliberate decision every day to increase flexibility. Tracy discovered the importance of flexibility and stretching during her solo 3,527-mile bicycle ride across the United States. Even though she burned over 10,000 calories daily without stretching, she wouldn't have been able to get on her bicycle the next morning.

The solution – Daily stretching!

Yoga and Pilates are great tools. It's never too late. The lesson here is stretch daily and never stop!

Regular Exercise

For some, that's a dirty word, but not us.

Exercise is a structured, planned activity to improve the physical conditioning of any part of your body.

Focusing the effort on strengthening your muscles is critical for overall good health. Remember, the heart is a muscle too, and for living a longer, healthier life, this must be a strong muscle. Your life may depend on it.

In this era, we don't get the physical activity our ancestors did. The human body should not sit in front of computers all day, spend three hours sitting on a couch in front of a TV, and then go to bed. Unless your job keeps you moving all day, you probably need to get some sort of exercise and movement scheduled throughout the day.

Exercise can reverse numerous age-related changes in your bones, joints, and muscles. It's never too late to start living a healthy and more active life. Once you see the difference it makes in your life like it did in ours, it will hook you.

Research is showing that exercise can help strengthen your bones while reducing the rate of bone loss. Increased physical activity will help delay the progression of osteoporosis because activity slows bone loss. Weight-bearing exercise is usually overlooked but is critical for longevity and bone health. Brisk walking, stair climbing, hiking, dancing, jogging, jumping rope, and tennis are examples of weight-bearing exercises to consider. Anything that has your body working against gravity is good for strength training.

Let's not use age as an excuse! Growing older, you can increase your strength and muscle mass through exercise.

The National Council of Aging[2] found that every 11 seconds, an adult over the age of 65 visits the emergency room for a fall. The statics are even more frightening when you consider that an older adult dies every 19 minutes from a fall. Tracy's beloved grandfather is one of these statistics. Take this seriously because it's a real issue. Yoga and tai chi can help with balance and coordination, which reduces fall risks. For more information on exercise see Chapter 19.

> *"Those who think they have no time for bodily exercise will sooner or later have to find time for illness."*
>
> Edward Stanley

Fighting Inflammation

One of the key contributors to the joint aches and pains of aging is inflammation.

White blood cells protect you from infections, viruses, and is key to fighting these issues. But in certain diseases like arthritis, your immune system thinks it is fighting off foreign invaders when there are none. When this damages your protective structure, it often leads to autoimmune diseases. When the body thinks healthy cells are bad, the body responds negatively.

Common issues caused by inflammation:

- Asthma
- Tuberculosis
- Periodontitis
- Crohn's disease
- Sinusitis
- Chronic Peptic Ulcer
- Rheumatoid Arthritis

Inflammaging

One study[3] calls it "inflammaging," a condition where blood inflammation markers indicate increased susceptibility to chronic disability, frailty, and premature death. The study also implicates "inflammaging" in the following:

- Cardiovascular diseases
- Chronic kidney disease
- Type 2 diabetes
- Depression
- Frailty
- Decline of cognitive function

Alzheimer's disease was implicated in a study[4] with 3,130 participants. It concluded systemic infection and inflammation are typical for the elderly and is critical to get the immune system back to normal to prevent the risk of developing Alzheimer's.

What's the Best way to Fight Inflammation?

Start with an anti-inflammatory diet.

Here's a list of foods known to increase inflammation, which is contrary to aging and better health:

- White bread
- Deep-Fried foods especially in omega-6 oil
- Sugar and High-Fructose Corn Syrup
- Deli Meat and Bacon
- Processed foods
- Excessive alcohol

Choose longevity healthy foods which helps to fight inflammation:

- Tomatoes
- Extra Virgin Olive Oil
- Green leafy vegetables, such as spinach, kale, and collards
- Nuts like almonds and walnuts
- Fatty fish like salmon, mackerel, tuna, and sardines
- Broccoli
- Avocados
- Dark Chocolate and Cocoa
- Berries which are low glycemic and are a healthy choice because of the polyphenols
  - Blueberries
  - Raspberries
  - Blackberries

www.LongevityCodes.com

- - Strawberries
  - Cherries
- Green Tea
- Peppers

If you're suffering from aches and pains, it may not be because of aging. Look closely at your diet and how it might be contributing to the issue.

Supplements Help

Fred has seen great results in reducing his aches and pains with supplements. Once he started eating foods that help him and not harm him, the weight started coming off, which gave him more energy while reducing his pain. Since eating the perfect diet is overwhelming, supplementation can help.

There are some specific supplements to consider when dealing with chronic pain.

Redox Signaling Molecules has helped almost eliminate Fred's knee pain.

Learn more at: *www.Longevitycodes.com/redox*

Be sure to check with your doctor before adding any supplements because they may cause an adverse reaction to medication and before starting an exercise program.

Consider these potent anti-inflammatory properties:

Turmeric and Curcumin

The turmeric root is known for its abundant anti-inflammatory properties. Curcumin is the active ingredient in turmeric and only makes up about 3% of it, which is why curcumin supplementation makes sense. Research studies have proven turmeric and curcumin are more effective than most common over the counter pain medications. We take a curcumin supplement daily to help fight chronic inflammation. Curcumin is more effective when combined with black pepper for the most significant health benefits.

Ginger

Ginger is another remarkable root for fighting pain and inflammation. Ginger can be freshly ground or found as a supplement in capsule form. We put fresh ginger in our morning green protein shake. Those who take blood-thinning medications must avoid ginger.

Omega-3

Fish oil and their healthy omega-3 fatty acids are also beneficial for joints and overall health. If you don't like salmon, mackerel, and other healthy fish, or you don't eat them regularly, then fish oil supplements are worth considering. Krill oil supplements are also highly anti-inflammatory, and some believed better absorbed in the body.

Glucosamine and Chondroitin Sulfate

Glucosamine and chondroitin sulfate are well known for helping with arthritis pain by fighting inflammation. It promotes cartilage formation and repair. The vitamin section

www.LongevityCodes.com

has many different formulas to choose from, but be careful and purchase high quality and see how it helps you.

You cannot allow negative thinking and believing that aches and pains of aging are the norm.

Here's your first line of defense:

- Get to and remain at a healthy weight
- Focus on flexibility
- Exercise regularly
- Eliminate inflammatory foods
- Add anti-inflammatory foods
- Supplement as needed

Chronic pain does not have to be an inevitable result of aging. You can do something

Get additional FREE RESOURCES at
www.LongevityCodes.com

www.LongevityCodes.com

Chapter 13

Overcome Setbacks

"Acceptance of what has happened is the first step to overcoming the consequences of any misfortune."
William James

Setbacks are a part of life, and how you respond separates the successful from the unsuccessful.

Tracy learned the importance of overcoming setbacks at the age of 17. A few weeks after leaving the hospital with a diagnosis of diabetes, she and her friends went to the movie theater. Remembering she could not have anything to eat or drink, she asked the concession stand clerk for a cup so she could get a drink out of the water fountain. It's hard to imagine something like this happening now, but this was before diet soft drinks and bottled water. The clerk refused, and Tracy fled the theater in tears asking, "why me?" This was a pivotal moment in Tracy's life as her setbacks outweighed her ability to deal with them. While lying in bed sobbing for several hours, she came to a fork in the road and said, "Tracy you have two choices, you can be better or bitter, which one will you choose?" At that moment, she chose to be better and started her journey of overcoming setbacks.

What should you do when setbacks occur?

www.LongevityCodes.com
___

DO

Expect them
- Setbacks happen and are a normal part of life, so expect them.
- When setbacks happen, it's essential to have a plan of action before they occur.
- When mentally prepared to deal with setbacks, you won't be caught unaware.

Forgive yourself and eliminate blame.
- Didn't have the healthiest meal last night? You cannot beat yourself up. Start fresh again NOW do not wait until tomorrow.
- Blame doesn't motivate change; forgiveness does.
- Focus on goals, and your WHY keeps you from feeling overwhelmed by blame.

Set a time limit for self-pity
- Each person is different. The severity of the setback impacts how much time is allowed for self-pity.
- No matter the situation, set a time and date when to stop and move on.

Get help
- If stuck and having trouble overcoming the setback, ask for help.
- Start by sharing challenges with friends or family who are empathetic and encouraging.
- Need extra help? Get a coach who walks the walk already and understand the struggles.

Just the facts and remove emotion.
- Eliminate the "I've always made this mistake" mindset.

- The common problem is to catastrophize the situation and make it even worse. Look at the situation as objectively as possible.
- A third party helps to provide a different viewpoint.

Think about the future and less about what went wrong
- Tomorrow is a new day with new possibilities.
- Projecting the future benefits of current actions will help maintain positive changes.

Give yourself enough time.
- Do not expect to overcome setbacks instantly.
- Be realistic, and don't lose hope.

The long-term perspective
- Think of it from a long-term perspective. Something stressful today probably won't matter in ten years. Will it seem huge then?
- Measure life by its entirety, not by current setbacks or failures.

Get plenty of rest.
- Lack of sleep aggravates depression and loss of energy.
- Restful sleep helps to stay the course.
- Disruptive sleep impairs judgment.

DON'T

Relapse
- Stay the course
- Do not look back

Do not allow negative self-talk.

- Do not listen to your inner critic because it can overwhelm thoughts.
- Write down positive affirmations and speak them out loud several times a day.
- The more negative thoughts, the more it is believed. The reverse is true. The more positive thoughts, the more it's internalized.

Vent appropriately
- Don't relieve stress with overeating, drinking, or other unhealthy behaviors.
- Share frustrations with positive individuals who have the same healthy belief system.

Everyone has struggles in their life, health, business, relationships, and families. Learning how to accept struggles and setbacks is what helps you become better. When setbacks happen, and they will, it is crucial to have a plan of action in place before obstacles occur.

What setbacks derail your health and longevity journey?

Do not allow fear, doubt or self-sabotage keep you from overcoming setbacks.

Chapter 14

The Secret to More Energy

Mitochondria are energy powerplants in the cells, playing a critical role in life and health. The bottom line, they convert oxygen and nutrients into ATP, which is the primary energy-carrying molecule for most of your cellular processes. Muscles, especially the heart muscle, have the most mitochondria. Some cells can have thousands, and others have very few depending on energy needs. When the mitochondria are not functioning correctly, serious health issues arise.

One study[1] stated that impaired mitochondrial function (sometimes called mitochondria dysfunction) causes neurodegenerative diseases like Alzheimer's and Parkinson's, along with its role in the aging process.

What do you do to protect them?

When you improve the health of your cells, it helps the mitochondria.

Improving the strength and performance of this crucial player impacts health and longevity.

Move

Need another reason to exercise? Physical activity, especially High-Intensity Interval Training, boosts mitochondria production and increases the size and number of mitochondria in your muscles.

Feed the Mitochondria

Mitochondria creates ATP from fatty acids or carbohydrates. Energy produced from burning fats reduces the production of free radicals, which is a good thing. Healthy foods for mitochondria health are wild-caught fish, extra virgin olive oil, avocados, pasture-raised meat, nuts, and seeds.

Sunshine

Sunshine converts into Vitamin D, which also boosts mitochondria production. Ask your doctor for a Vitamin D blood test to check your levels. Most people are deficient in this critical vitamin because of the lack of sun exposure. Fear of skin cancer causes many to avoid the sun and become low in this crucial vitamin. Avoid getting a sunburn to reduce the risk of skin damage.

Intermittent Fasting

Increasing autophagy by intermittent fasting, which removes unhealthy and damaged cells, is a longevity approach. Eliminating these cells will help reduce mitochondrial free radical production and improve mitochondria health.

Quality Sleep

During sleep, the brain removes waste products and preserves mitochondria. Sleep is critical for cellular health! Strive for seven to eight hours of high-quality sleep nightly. Think of this as a "Spa Day" for your brain.

Cold Exposure

Shocking the body with a quick burst of cold temperature puts the body in survival mode, which revs up mitochondrial production. To shock your body, try 30-seconds of a chilly blast of water at the end of the shower. Or consider walking outside in the winter with just a T-shirt on. Want to go to the extreme? Jump in a cryotherapy tank for a few minutes at 200° below zero (Fahrenheit) for a quick shock to the mitochondria.

Eat Low Glycemic

Eating sugar or high carb foods that quickly convert to sugar, causes inflammation which is terrible for the mitochondria. As much as possible, stay away from processed foods and eat low carb meals which doesn't spike the blood sugar.

Supplement

It is almost impossible to get all the nutrients you need from diet alone. Supplementation can improve cellular health and boost mitochondria.

Here's a few supplements to consider for mitochondria health:

- Magnesium
- Fish or krill oil
- CoQ10
- Glutathione
- L-Carnitine
- Alpha Lipoic Acid

www.LongevityCodes.com

Your mitochondria must be functioning optimally to be genuinely healthy.

An important longevity codes strategy to think about daily is:

> ***Will this help or hurt my mitochondria?***

Check out
LONGEVITY CODES COACHING PROGRAM
www.LongevityCodes.com
Our **Longevity Codes Certified Coach** will help you implement the principles in this book and provide the tools and accountability you need to achieve fast results.

Chapter 15

Strategies for Better Gut Health

It's 1907 Paris, France and you have a stomachache. Because of the intense discomfort, you visit your friend Élie Metchnikoff, who happens to be a Russian Nobel laureate scientist. What does he suggest? Drink a cup of sour milk fermented with bacteria. It sounds nasty, but it became the rage with doctors prescribing the sour milk diet to their patients. Metchnikoff was early in understanding the correlation between bacteria in the gut and health.

Gut health is now becoming a hot topic. Commercials touting the importance of probiotics are everywhere, and it is a generally accepted conversation.

Here you are armed with the latest information and research on probiotics. If you are unsure about probiotics, take this chapter and show your physician the connection between gut health and living longer. Since we believe in having a healthy immune system, this is something we take seriously and is why we rarely get sick.

What's gut bacteria?

The body has between 300 and 500 types of bacteria living in the gut. Viruses, fungi, and bacteria create what is called the microbiota. Sometimes referred to as the microbiome.

Each person has a unique microbiota, which is partly determined at birth but can change with diet and lifestyle. Bacteria live throughout the body, but your overall health is determined mainly by the bacteria that line the digestive system.

Bacteria live in the digestive system and live predominately in the intestines and colon. The gut microbiota helps to digest food that is impossible for your stomach to digest otherwise. A healthy microbiome helps absorb nutrition, builds immune cells, fights disease, improves sleep, boost metabolism, and improves the mood. If your gut is not healthy, it will lead to numerous serious diseases.

Interest peaked? Let's look at the science.

A study[1] conducted in Italy compared gut bacteria and microbiota of centenarians (age 100+) and supercentenarians (ages 110+). Researchers found common strains of bacteria in the gut of the supercentenarians that were unique. What remained undetermined was, did they have these strains throughout their life, or if somehow, they developed them later? Also, unclear is if these strains contributed to their longevity. Even though the study appears inconclusive, they believe health-associated gut bacteria is involved with what they call "longevity adaptation."

These findings give a compelling reason to focus on your gut health!

Since gut bacteria and gut health are critical for living a longer and healthier life, what are you going to do?

Take Probiotics

As mentioned earlier, we have been taking probiotic supplements for many years and believe in the benefits. Take high potency, multiple strain, and purchase high quality. Focusing on quality versus price is best.

Eat Fermented Foods

A good source of healthy bacteria for the gut is fermented foods. Examples are:
- Sauerkraut
- Kefir
- Kimchi
- Kombucha
- Fermented vegetables
- Miso

Reduce Stress

Stress impacts all health systems, including the gut. Remember the last time you were nervous or stressed to the point you were sick at your stomach? Case closed!

Stressors are known to affect gut health negatively, include:

- Psychological stress
- Environmental stress (things like extreme heat, cold, or noise)
- Sleep deprivation
- Disruption of the circadian rhythm

Eat Prebiotic Fiber

Probiotics need to feed on non-digestible carbohydrates, which are called prebiotics, which help beneficial gut bacteria grow and multiply. Examples are things like:

- Whole grains
- Garlic
- Asparagus
- Onions
- Bananas
- Artichokes

Get Enough Sleep

Studies have shown poor and disrupted sleep negatively impacts your gut health and increases inflammation.

Need help getting better quality sleep? Be sure to pay close attention to Chapter 21 and implement these strategies.

Eat Less Sugar and Artificial Sweeteners

Consuming an abundance of sugar and artificial sweeteners are toxic to the body. Researchers are finding that sugar and sweeteners create problems for the balance of the gut microbiome. Artificial sweeteners negatively impact blood glucose levels, which influences the gut flora.

Avoid Taking Antibiotics Unnecessarily

While antibiotics save lives, and sometimes you cannot avoid them, according to the CDC[2], 30% of antibiotics prescribed are unnecessary. Yes, they do kill the harmful bacteria, but unfortunately, they kill the good ones too. When antibiotics are needed, consider taking an extra probiotic to re-establish a better balance, but always check with your medical team first.

Exercise Regularly

Studies show that athletes have a wider variety of good gut flora than those who are sedentary. Want to live longer? Want to reduce the risk of developing certain diseases? Adding exercise to your daily routine is paramount. Your future self will thank you for it.

Consider a Vegetarian Diet

Some studies report that people who choose to eat a vegetarian diet have better gut bacteria than people who eat meat. One explanation could be because of the increased fiber in the vegetarian diet. Because of other research, we have not transitioned to a vegetarian lifestyle, but do have meatless days throughout the week. It appears that consuming less meat could positively impact longevity. Read how to find your longevity diet in Chapter 7.

Want to live a longer, healthier life? Start with the gut. The gut is often called "the second brain." Building a healthy gut microbiome is a critical longevity strategy.

www.LongevityCodes.com

Chapter 16

Taking Control of Your Health

"Only you can control your future."
Dr. Seuss

At the age of 50, Orville Rogers decided to take control of his health after reading Dr. Kenneth H Cooper's book "Running." What's the big deal? Mr. Rogers continued to set world records at the age of 100.

Today is the day to start taking control of your health.

If you are someone who thinks age is a limitation, remember Orville. Knowing your "WHY" is critical to start this process, but then keeping it up is another factor. Changing behavior boils down to a decision only you can make. Are you doing it because of external reasons like your spouse, doctor, or friend, wants you to get healthy? Those reasons will derail your transformation. For example, "I want to lose 20 pounds because I'm going to a reunion and want to look fabulous." Or "my doctor is on my case about lowering my blood pressure, and I'm tired of it." While those reasons will help you start initially, they will not help maintain the change needed for good health.

Decide to live longer for internal reasons like "I want to watch my kids and grandkids grow up" or "I want to be healthier and have more energy." Thoughts like these help you make appropriate changes and maintain healthy behaviors.

www.LongevityCodes.com

Remember reaching and maintaining health goals is a marathon and NOT a sprint!

Tips for taking control of your health:

Write Down Goals
- Dr. Gail Matthews[1] discovered that those who wrote down their goals regularly were 42% more likely to achieve them.

Enter it on the Calendar
- Do you cancel the necessary meetings on your calendar? Probably not! Let's treat health, like other vital activities.

Ask for Help
- It's okay and healthy to ask for help when struggling.

Get Quality Sleep
- Remember to go to bed and wake up at about the same time each day, even on weekends.
- Stop watching TV or using electronic devices at least an hour before bedtime.
- Keep the bedroom cold and dark.

Do Not Smoke
- If you do, find a way to stop. Your future self will thank you!

www.LongevityCodes.com

Meditate
- Start in a dimly lit room and sit in a straight-back chair with both feet on the floor, take five or six deep breaths.
- Begin breathing normally. Focus attention on breathing, inhale through nose, exhale through mouth. Let everything else go.
- Five minutes is all it takes to achieve benefits, but 20 minutes is even better.
- The nice thing with meditation is NO JUDGEMENT. If your mind wanders, go back to focusing on breathing.

Remove negative influences
- Write down everything negative on a piece of paper and then burn it. Once you have tried this, you'll be amazed at how this symbolizes those negative things leaving your life.
- Reduce time spent watching or listening to negative things.
- Spend less time with negative people.

Stay organized
- Plan healthy meals or snacks before being tempted.
- Set out workout clothes the night before.

Enroll in a class
- Learn a new hobby.
- Read something inspirational.

www.LongevityCodes.com

Hydrate
- Human bodies consist of 60% water.
- Water removes toxins from the body.
- Drink pure filtered water if possible.
- Hunger may be a sign of dehydration. Drink a glass of water and wait 15 minutes to see if hunger subsides.

Volunteering
- Helping others promotes a longer life.
- It helps decrease depression and reduces stress.

Do not try to change everything at once. Small changes equal significant results over time. Just like Tracy's bicycle ride across the United States, every day she peddled closer to New York City. She did not leave San Francisco, saying, "oh, I have 3,527 miles until I reach the Brooklyn Bridge." Instead, she said, "I'm going for a bike ride." Even small daily steps towards your goal over time will yield significant results.

You CAN take control of your health!

Chapter 17

The Master Antioxidant

Glutathione is "The Master Antioxidant" because it's essential for anti-aging, cellular health, and longevity. It's found in every cell, including plants, animals, and has three types of amino acid molecules:

- Cysteine
- Glycine
- Glutamic acid (or glutamate)

The combination of these three amino acids helps to detox by removing free radicals, toxins, and heavy metals.

What's unique about glutathione, unlike most antioxidants, is the body produces it in the liver. The body's ability to provide an adequate amount of glutathione reduces as you age. Stress, infections, toxins, unhealthy diets, pollution, radiation, along with medications, can all deplete glutathione.

Why is glutathione so important? Glutathione plays a vital role in several critical areas:

- Supports the immune function
- Fights oxidative stress from free radicals
- Assists programmed cell death known as apoptosis
- Lowers inflammation
- Improves mental health
- Protects the brain
- Fights infections

- Improves gut health
- Helps with heart health
- Improves kidney health
- Protects the liver
- Lungs & airways
- Skin health
- Eye health

See why your longevity strategy needs to include glutathione?

The focal point of this chapter is the following three essentials for better health:

1. Fights Oxidative Stress
2. Boosts Immune Function
3. Lowers Inflammation

Oxidative Stress

Glutathione helps to reduce ROS and oxidative stress that damages the DNA and cells.

The mitochondria primarily produce ROS in cells, which creates more than the cells can remove. Reinforcements of antioxidants come to the rescue to handle the overproduction. Glutathione peroxidase is the principal ROS fighter.

A Study[1] linked oxidative stress to these diseases:

- Alzheimer's disease
- Parkinson's disease
- Cancer
- Diabetes

- High blood pressure
- Atherosclerosis
- Stroke
- Inflammatory disorders
- Chronic fatigue syndrome
- Asthma

Glutathione plays a pivotal role in reducing oxidative stress.

Immune System

Without enough glutathione, your immune cells cannot fight infections. One study[2] showed that glutathione helped to control the growth of tuberculosis. According to the World Health Organization[3], in 2018, 1.5 million people died from tuberculosis.

Low Glutathione levels can lead to higher rates of infections. Many chronic diseases weaken the immune system.

Lowers Inflammation

Glutathione can block the production of inflammatory cytokines. Why should you block cytokines? Because they can keep you at a state of constant low-grade inflammation.

Inflammation can cause:

- Rheumatoid arthritis
- Asthma
- Sinusitis
- Chronic peptic ulcer
- Tuberculosis

- Ulcerative colitis and Crohn's disease
- Periodontitis
- Active hepatitis

How to Boost Glutathione

Bob, a coaching client of Tracy's, asked, "Why not just take one of the glutathione supplements on the market and boost it that way?"

Not so fast! It turns out it's not that simple. Glutathione is a protein molecule quickly digested in the stomach, and only a small amount makes it to the bloodstream. If you decide to try a supplement, make sure their product has scientific backing and is effective.

The best way to increase glutathione levels is with an intravenous drip or injections. Consider this option if your levels are low and need to boost quickly. Depending on where you live, the price ranges between $100 and $200.

If you don't like needles boost naturally by choosing foods high in glutathione.

High sulfur foods and cruciferous vegetables:

- Garlic
- Onions
- Broccoli
- Cauliflower
- Cabbage
- Brussel sprouts

Other foods to consider:

- Avocados
- Potatoes
- Asparagus
- Peppers
- Squash
- Carrots
- Spinach
- Melons

Selenium helps to boost glutathione, and good sources are:

- Beef
- Organ meats
- Fish
- Sardines
- Chicken
- Brown rice
- Cottage cheese
- Brazil nuts
- Raw liver from organic grass-fed cows

Supplements are known to help:

- Turmeric extract
- Whey protein
- Vitamin C
- Vitamin E
- Zinc
- Magnesium
- N-acetyl cysteine (NAC)
- Alpha-lipoic acid
- Selenium
- Milk thistle

Sulfur Rich Foods

Sulfur is a significant mineral found in some protein and plant foods. Bodies need sulfur for the synthesis of glutathione.

Whey Protein

Glutathione requires the amino acid cysteine for synthesis. Whey protein is high in cysteine. Another study[4] reported that whey protein could increase glutathione levels, helping reduce oxidative stress. For years our morning ritual has included adding whey in our green protein shake.

Vitamin C

A critical go-to antioxidant that helps protect from oxidative stress and damage is Vitamin C. A 13-week study[5] had adults take 500-1000 mg of Vitamin C daily. Participants increased their white blood cells by 18%, which is vital for fighting infection. Another study[6] gave participants 500 mg per day and saw a 47% glutathione increase in the red blood cells. Increasing red blood cells is critical for carrying oxygen to the lungs and other organs.

Turmeric or Curcumin Extract

Consider supplementing with turmeric or curcumin extract to help lower inflammation. Studies[7] have shown that turmeric or curcumin extract could increase glutathione levels and possibly reduce cancer cells.

Other Methods to Boost Glutathione

Exercise

Want to live a longer, healthier life? Consider adding exercise for better heart health and boosting glutathione. A study[8] to determine the connection between physical activity and glutathione levels showed it increased glutathione along with other antioxidants.

What's interesting is combining weight training and cardio increases glutathione compared to doing them separately. In the past, the general rule was to practice these exercises on different days.

But don't overdo it! One study[9] showed athletes who didn't get adequate rest and nutrition, in combination with overtraining, decreased their glutathione production.

Alcohol

Excessive alcohol can deplete the glutathione level in the lungs. When lungs are healthy, they have approximately 1,000 times the glutathione of other parts of the body. Researchers[10] found those who regularly consume excessive amounts of alcohol had up to a 90% decrease in lung glutathione levels. One more reason to cut back or eliminate alcohol.

Sleep

Having a restful night's sleep is paramount in maintaining a healthy glutathione level. Research shows people who don't get enough sleep regularly have decreased glutathione.

According to one study, [11] comparing healthy adults to a group of people with insomnia, found much lower glutathione levels in the insomnia group.

Do glutathione levels need to be tested?

Do you suffer from any of these?

- Lack of energy and tired all the time
- Brain fog
- Muscle and joint pain
- Problems sleeping

If so, it could be an indication of low glutathione levels.

Consider talking to your doctor about having your levels checked. If your levels are low, practice some of these strategies.

Glutathione is another crucial tool in your quest to live a longer, healthier life.

Check out
LONGEVITY CODES COACHING PROGRAM
www.LongevityCodes.com
Our **Longevity Codes Certified Coach** will help you implement the principles in this book and provide the tools and accountability you need to achieve fast results.

Chapter 18

Save Money While Living Longer

What if you could save money, lose weight, prevent Type 2 diabetes, reduce the risk of certain cancers, and improve cellular health with one simple strategy?

What is it?

Fasting

It's easy! There's nothing to buy, no program to join, no counting, and you don't eat for a set period.

Most major religions practice fasting, and it has been around for thousands of years.

In 2016 the Nobel Prize in Physiology or Medicine was awarded to Yoshinori Ohsumi of the Tokyo Institute of Technology[1]. He discovered the mechanisms underlying autophagy, the fundamental process in which cells degrade, recycle, and repair themselves. Ohsumi was able to get a deeper understanding by experimenting on yeast and identified the mechanisms that also applied to the human cell.

What is Autophagy? The name comes from two Greek words: auto for self and phagy means eating. It means self-eating or self-devouring. That may sound disgusting, but it is merely the body's process of cleaning out damaged cells so they can regenerate with new healthy cells. Did you know you have a self-cleaning recycling system? Although that statement does make us laugh, it is incredible how important this recycling process is.

What does this have to do with fasting? Ohsumi found that by starving the cell, it forces it to either get stronger, die, or rebuild a new cell.

Jason Fung, M.D., first taught us the benefits of fasting. His work helps hundreds of patients with Type 2 Diabetes lower or eliminate their need for medications using fasting as the primary protocol. Dr. Fung's book *The Complete Guide to Fasting* provides a wealth of information with resources, verified, and detailed evidence on this protocol.

Thomas Seyfried, Ph.D., is a cancer expert and suggests a yearly seven-day water-only fast. He believes it can help remove cancer cells, therefore preventing cancer.

What do you think, could an annual seven-day water only fast be a longevity strategy for preventing cancer? We both do a weekly 24-hour fast, and even though it was hard at first, we now look forward to it. Fred has done several 48-hour fasts and plans to make an annual seven-day fast part of his longevity strategy. Tracy must be more careful with multi-day fasting because of her Type 1 diabetes.

For several years' researchers have been studying fasting and have found a common theme. One of the problems with the epidemic rise of obesity is the abundance of food at your disposal. Having three square meals a day and snacks in between is a recent development in human history. Until a few hundred years ago, food was not as plentiful as it is now. Our ancestors lived in a feast or famine state. Some experts suggest that eating throughout the day is useful for keeping blood sugars level. Still, for cellular health, this reasoning is flawed.

The Paleo movement suggests the human body cannot handle all the chemicals and processed foods consumed today in the Western diet. We could not agree more! There is some logic behind the Paleo concept of only eating what a cave dweller would eat, but this is often hard to manage. It's a good strategy since it keeps you from eating so many unhealthy processed foods. Consuming large amounts of sugar, high fructose corn syrup, and unhealthy hydrogenated oils hurt your body.

Taking the caveman's approach to fasting makes sense. They did not eat three square meals a day, along with snacking and often went days without eating.

Fasting is still practiced in many religions today, just like it was in ancient times.

Fasting is a normal part of the human experience, and science is now able to back up this practice with research on how valuable it is for your cellular health.

Top 10 reasons to implement Intermittent Fasting as one of your Longevity Codes strategies:

1. It can help you live longer by slowing down the aging process
2. Helps to protect against cancer (as mentioned earlier)
3. Helps with weight loss (this makes sense unless after a fast you eat an abundance of unhealthy processed foods to make up for it)
4. Improves heart health and blood pressure
5. Reduced insulin resistance or risk of developing Type 2 diabetes
6. Reduce oxidative stress and inflammation
7. Assists with cellular repair (see above section on autophagy)

8. Improves mental acuity and brain function
9. May help prevent Alzheimer's disease
10. Some evidence is now showing it may help with Parkinson's disease

Common types of fasting:

- **The Circadian Rhythm Fast** – This mimics your body's natural clock by fasting after sunset to sunrise (approximately 13 hours long).
- **16 Hour Fast** with eight-hour eating window – Hugh Jackson made this famous as a quick way to remove access weight.
- **18 Hour Fast** with six hours to eat – this type of fast helps the liver remove more glycogen, helps your body use ketones for fuel while helping your body remove cells that are damaged.
- **The 5:2 Eating Plan** – Eat regularly for five days, and the remaining two days restrict caloric intake to 500 calories for women and 600 for men.
- **Fasting Mimicking Diet**[2] – Reduced calories for five days with a 50/50 ratio of complex carbs to healthy fats. For overall good health, practice this once or twice a year. If you have health issues or need to lose a significant amount of weight, this system can be done once a month for numerous months, depending on your risk factors.
- **24 Hour Fast** is simple, don't eat or drink anything with calories for 24 hours. A 24 hour fast is the one we practice most weeks. Fred prefers to fast from dinner to dinner, and Tracy prefers breakfast to breakfast.
- **Dinner to Break (fast)** with no snacking and drinking only water or herbal tea. Not eating after

dinner is probably what you grew up doing. Only on rare occasions did people ever snack after eating dinner.
- **48 Hour Fast** is useful for reaching autophagy. Fred has completed several 48-hour fasts and likes this strategy.
- **Multi 3-5 Day Fasts** – Siim Land says he practices a three to five day fast once a quarter. He believes that after five days, the value decreases unless you need a specific result like reducing a cancerous tumor or other therapeutic reasons.

Land likes to break his fasts slowly with drinking water with lemon, sliced ginger, and a couple of teaspoons of apple cider vinegar. He mentions this wakes up the stomach and prepares it better to start ingesting food. He also suggests starting with some fermented foods with healthy probiotics to help aid digestion. Land also suggests a day or two before starting a multi-day fast, eat a ketogenic diet.

The list of fasts could go on and on, but consider the fast based on the results you need.

We're all different. What works best for us may not work best for you.

When we first started fasting, the struggle was real. Fred was one of those people always thinking about what he was going to eat next. He was terrified to experience hunger. Because of this fear, he felt that it must have been some deep-rooted psychological issue. Fasting has helped him remember the importance of having the right mindset, and skipping a few meals would not hurt him but was freeing. Tracy, on the other hand, was never able to experiment with fasting until she started using an insulin pump and Continuous Glucose

Monitor. Her focus on food was always in relationship to blood sugar management. Tracy understood that if during a fast, she felt hungry, and her blood glucose levels were normal, then it was a mindset issue. When this occurs, she drinks more water and uses positive affirmations to help ease the hunger pain.

The benefits of fasting are clear but counter to decades of marketing, advertising, and especially TV commercials. Autophagy helps with longevity and improves with fasting. The research on how human cells work is advancing, and we will continue to research and share as it relates to health and longevity.

Scientific research and studies support intermittent fasting to live a longer, healthier life.

Before deciding on trying one of these fasts, check with your doctor first. Certain medications and health conditions may cause harmful effects during a fast. Do your research, and if your physician gives you the go-ahead, give it a try. Again, if you have any health issues, you **must** check with your doctor first. Don't be surprised if your physician hasn't heard of the medical benefits of fasting because it's not taught in medical school. Explaining to your doctor the benefits and the research will open their eyes to a possible new treatment plan.

Get additional FREE RESOURCES at

www.LongevityCodes.com

Chapter 19

Move for Life

"We do not stop exercising because we grow old - we grow old because we stop exercising."
Kenneth Cooper, MD (Father of Aerobics)

Tracy's grandmother Mary lived to be 99 years old and died quickly from pneumonia. Once she stopped driving, her answer to that challenge was buying herself an adult three-wheel bicycle, which she rode to the grocery store daily. The patriarch of the family was a role model to her community. One story shared decades after her death was how she was able to do the splits even at the age of 90. Her love of horses kept her active, and she rode daily even in her late 90s. What an example of how daily movement is critical for living a longer, healthier life—notice we did not use the word exercise but replaced it with the positive word "movement." Mary was a great example of how moving kept her young and sharp.

Don't stop reading this chapter because of guilt or thinking, "I can't exercise!" Nor is this a call to ride your bicycle across the United States like Tracy did, but how to find movement in daily life.

It is essential to check with your doctor before starting a fitness program. The reason this is so critical is you want to make sure there aren't any underlying medical issues. Certain medications have adverse reactions impacted by exercise too.

According to a study[1] tracking the activity levels of 1,274 men over five years found every extra 30 minutes of light activity reduced the chance of death by 15%. Participants who practiced at least 150 minutes a week of moderate to vigorous exercise were approximately 40% less likely to die during the study. The results remained the same whether the physical activity was less than 10 minutes or more than 10 minutes. Based on this study, you can't use the excuse "I don't have time to exercise."

Leisure activities lowers the risk of death for all causes, including cancer and cardiovascular disease, based on a study[2] of 88,140 United States adults.

If we cited every scientific peer-reviewed research on the importance of exercise, this book would take decades to read. Getting daily movement in your life is a longevity strategy you won't want to ignore.

What's the best type of exercise? The one you do! All joking aside, they all have different benefits but don't stick with just one. Find something you enjoy because you'll continue to do it.

Walking

Don't overlook the importance of walking. People think to be healthy; you need to be a long-distance runner, triathlete, weightlifter, or workout every day at the gym. Obviously, this isn't true! When Tracy first works with a new coaching client, they are shocked when she merely suggests starting a walking program. Their first reaction is always; it can't be that simple. But it really is!

<www.LongevityCodes.com>

Meeting "Sally" in Sacramento, California, on the third day of Tracy's solo 3,527-mile bicycle ride across the United States, was life-changing for both of them. Waiting for the light to turn green, Tracy noticed Sally getting off the bus and struggling to make it to the bus stop seat. Sally said, "I wish I could ride my bicycle across the city." Tracy proceeded to tell her she was riding her bicycle to New York City*. Feeling the need to encourage Sally, Tracy got off the bike, climbed up the curb, and started chatting with her. She was waiting for a ride because she couldn't walk the block or two to her house. Sally was in her mid-30s, pleasant, without hope, and morbidly obese. The coach in Tracy came out, and she started asking her questions about what she could do. Tracy asked, "Can you walk to the end of your street?" "Can you walk next door?" All Tracy wanted to do was help her walk home from the bus stop. Every answer to these questions was the same, "I can't." Tracy's final question was, "can you walk to the end of your driveway?" She said, "I think I can!" Yes, music to Tracy's ears because Sally had a glimmer of hope. Tracy quickly helped her develop a plan, made sure it was doable, had no questions, and off Tracy went on her bicycle. As Tracy was finishing her ride, she received a message from Sally saying she had just signed up for her first 5k walk. That's 3.1 miles for someone who couldn't even walk a block several months earlier. This strategy works and hang on tight as you learn about the power of walking.

* If you would like to watch a short 3-minute recap of Tracy's bicycle ride across the country go to https://www.tracyherbert.com/

"Walking is man's best medicine."
Hippocrates

Benefits of Walking

Cancer Risk Reduction

An American Cancer Society study[3] found women who walked seven hours or more a week had a 14% lower risk of developing breast cancer. What's exciting is this study found walking also protected women who are overweight, who typically have an increased risk of developing breast cancer.

Reduced Risk of Diabetes

The American Diabetes Association[4] found that walking lowers blood sugar levels and lowers the risk of developing diabetes. The study reported regular physical activity also lowers A1c.

Improves Heart Health

Frequently walking lowers blood pressure by as much as 11% and reduces the risk of stroke by 20-40%.

People who walk at a moderate pace for at least 30 minutes, five or more days per week, had a 30% lower risk of cardiovascular disease than those who didn't walk.

Immune Function

During cold and flu season, those who walked at least 20 minutes most days of the week were 43% more likely to have fewer sick days. And those who were ill, the severity of the symptoms was less severe, and they experienced a shorter duration.

Brain Function

According to the National Council on Aging, those over the age of 60 who walked 45 minutes every day at a 16-minute mile pace greatly improved their cognitive performance. Those who walked 40 minutes three times a week slowed the age-related normal shrinking of the hippocampus. The hippocampus is the part of the brain associated with short-term memory. It is the first area of the brain to be damaged by Alzheimer's.

Your mood improves by walking. When you walk, your endorphins increase, enhancing your mood. When you walk for 20 minutes at a quick pace, your disposition can improve for 12 hours afterward.

Joint Pain

Walking helps reduce joint pain, even arthritis. People who walk five to six miles a week can prevent arthritis if you don't have arthritis start walking now. When walking, your muscles strengthen, and your joints are lubricated. Walking protects hips and knees, just the opposite of what so many people think. Remember, a good pair of shoes is critical to protect your knees, hips, and back.

Need help starting a walking program?

Always check with your doctor before starting an exercise program.

Walk as often as possible. You know the importance of exercising 30 minutes daily. Don't have time? Break it down to three 10-minute sessions, two 15-minute sessions, or one 30-minute session.

If you are like Tracy's friend Sally, mentioned earlier, for her walking 10 minutes was impossible. But today is a different story. Do what works best for you! Even if it's walking to the end of your driveway, it will improve your health. Many smartwatches or pedometers can help with step counting. Use one of these tools on an average day and see how many steps you take. Continue to add steps each day until you reach 10,000 steps (which is about 5 miles) or if you want to lose weight have a goal of 15,000 (which is a little over 7 miles) steps daily.

Metabolic Syndrome

Metabolic syndrome is a cluster of risk factors, abnormal cholesterol or triglyceride levels, increased blood pressure, elevated blood sugar, and extra body fat around the waist.

Go the extra mile, or at least 5,000 additional steps. A study[5] conducted at the University of Warwick found that having 15,000 steps per day can lead to far superior benefits. The study concluded those taking an extra 5,000 steps every day had no risk factors of metabolic syndrome.

Walking Tips

Walk faster for improved health. Those who walk more swiftly, even with fewer steps, have the same positive health outcomes as a healthy Body Mass Index (BMI) and waist circumference.

While warming up, walk at a slower pace, then quicken the pace and start walking like you're late to a meeting, then slow back down but keep walking. Repeat these steps the entire walk. After a few weeks, it's surprising how much more distance is covered when using this strategy. If you're a goal-setter, try walking 100 steps per minute or even faster.

Remember to build up slowly, especially if you haven't exercised in a while. A goal might be to walk about three miles in 45 minutes.

Having good posture is critical. Don't forget to swing your arms when walking—moving your arms opposite to how the legs are moving helps. You can add hand weights if you want but start at a low weight to make sure you can tolerate it. Never use leg weights when walking.

Several people we know use walking poles. It may provide extra security from the fear of falling, helps you get in shape for hiking, and builds arm strength.

Be sure to get proper fitting shoes. Having good shoes prevents injuries and helps protect your knees and hips. When wearing new shoes, be sure to pay attention to your feet to avoid developing blisters.

If the weather is too hot or too cold to walk, find a mall or other location that allows walkers.

Additional benefits of Walking

1. Burn calories
2. Strengthens the heart
3. Can help lower blood sugar
4. Eases joint pain
5. Boosts immune function
6. Increases energy
7. Improves mood
8. Extends life
9. Tones legs
10. Improves creative thinking

"The best kind of exercise is the ONE YOU DO!"
Tracy Herbert

High-Intensity Interval Training

What is High-Intensity Interval Training (HIIT)? This type of training is simple. The best way to describe this exercise is short bursts of energy with little downtime in between. When Tracy first researched HIIT, she thought it was too good to be true. How can you get all these benefits in such a short amount of time? As you age, your lung capacity decreases. The lung production benefits with this type of exercise and how it improves lung health as you age makes this a vital workout tool. Now, this is Tracy's favorite type of training, and she does it several times a week.

Benefits may include:

- Burns fat quicker
- Improves lung capacity
- Increases oxygen consumption

www.LongevityCodes.com

- Reduces heart rate
- Builds heart strength
- Improves blood pressure
- Burns a lot of calories in a short period (in less than 20 minutes per day)
- Increases metabolic rate
- Lowers Blood Sugar

Unfit but otherwise healthy middle-aged adults were able to improve their insulin sensitivity and blood sugar with this type of training three times per week for just two weeks. After only one training session, people with Type 2 diabetes were able to improve their blood sugar for the next 24 hours! Isn't that great news!

How to Perform HIIT

Check with your doctor before starting an exercise program.

1. Always warm up first. Start slowing for approximately 5-10 minutes.
2. Next, proceed with a burst of maximum effort for 30-45 seconds or as long as you can go, before slowing down. If you can talk or sing, you're not using enough energy. Make sure it's difficult but not impossible! The only competition is with yourself and not with a workout partner.
3. Slow down to bring the heart rate down for approximately 90 seconds and use less resistance if using a bicycle or elliptical machine.
4. Repeat the cycle of maximum effort and slow down cycle for three to six times, depending on your fitness level. If at first, you can only do one or two high-

intensity sessions, don't worry, you will get stronger over time if you stick with it. You want to alternate between short spurts of high-intensity exercise along with gentle recovery periods.
5. Cool down with a low-intensity version of the exercise you just performed for 5-10 minutes afterward. Don't skip this step, which helps reduce the risk of injury and improves heart rate recovery.
6. Stretching afterward is a perfect opportunity to stretch joints and muscles, which are already warm. Don't overdo it. Avoiding injury and improving flexibility is essential for longevity.

Ideas to Try:

- Walking or Running – One of Tracy's favorites is going to a local school track. Walk or run on the curves at a fast pace, then slow down on the straightaways. Once this becomes easy, switch and run or walk quickly on the straightaways and slow down on the curves. Neighborhood sidewalks work well. Watch out for uneven surfaces, which can lead to falls. Once Sally was able to walk to the end of her driveway, she started using this type of exercise to build up endurance while losing weight.
- Watching TV makes for an unusual exercise strategy – Walk or run in place during the show, and once a commercial comes on, increase intensity. No commercials? No problem! Use a 30-minute TV show and do interval training throughout the show and see how much better you feel.
- Bike riding – This was how Tracy built strength to ride her bicycle across the United States. Stationary

bikes work just as well. The same approach applies using bursts of high intensity with intervals of reduced intensity.
- Stairs - Find stairs and walk up and down to increase activity level. Walk up as fast as you can (safely) rest at the top for a about a minute and then walk down the stairs slowly. Repeat. Try to get in as many as you can in 20 minutes. In a short amount of time, you will see how quickly you have improved.
- Other exercises to try are swimming, pushups, jumping jacks, lunges, squats, jump rope, and weightlifting.

Remember to listen to your body – start with just a couple of intervals and SLOWLY increase the intensity as you get stronger.

Other Benefits of Exercise:

Studies prove that exercise lowers stress and depression. Mental health issues continue to rise in the United States, and having a prevention strategy like exercise provides hope without the adverse effects of medications. DO NOT STOP TAKING YOUR DEPRESSION MEDICATION, but check with your doctor about getting extra movement into your day.

Tai chi is a Chinese martial art that incorporates graceful movements that flow smoothly from one to the next. The centenarians of Okinawa live longer than most people in the world and practice Tai chi as part of their daily lives. The American Arthritis Foundation also recommends it for anyone experiencing arthritis joint pain. Tai chi helps people at all fitness levels. This unique exercise improves balance and promotes a positive mood.

A study[6] of older adults who practiced strength training at least twice a week had a 46% lower risk of death from any cause than those who did not do strength training. The sad thing is only 9.6% meet the twice a week guideline.

Yoga is another longevity strategy to consider. It improves flexibility, balance, strength, and reduces stress.

Tips

- Don't forget the water! Drinking water before, during, and after exercise, keeps you hydrated.
- Wait approximately 30 minutes after eating for gentle exercise and wait longer about two hours if doing something more strenuous.
- Set goals and stick with it.
- Don't overdo ANY exercise program. Remember, this is a marathon and not a sprint. If you start off to fast, it could lead to injury and burnout.
- Immediately stop exercising if something hurts and learn to listen to your body.
- Schedule the time you plan to exercise and block it on your calendar. You do not cancel important meetings, social events with friends, or time with family, shouldn't your health be the same?
- Swimming is often called the perfect workout. Water supports your body and takes the strain off joints.
- Keep a journal! Writing things down will give you a peek to how you are feeling

- Get a dog! Studies show that having a dog helps increase physical activity.
- Remember being a kid and receiving a star on your schoolwork? Use the same strategy and place a star on a calendar every day you exercise. The visualization will help encourage and challenge you to stay on task.
- Walk to a coworker's office instead of sending an email.
- When talking on the phone, stand up and walk around.
- Use a standing desk if possible. If not, set a timer and get up every 45 minutes while sitting, especially working or watching TV.
- Walk with a group of friends, family, or coworkers. It's more fun, and you'll have people to help you stay accountable.
- Suggest a walking meeting at work.
- Don't fear the hills. Walking up a steep hill provides additional benefits in less time.
- Set a goal that is difficult to reach but attainable.
- Expect setbacks and have an action plan before being tempted to skip exercise.

Accountability

Find a friend or accountability partner to help you stay on track. Two is always better than one! Many of Tracy's clients only need someone to help them stay accountable or to give them a friendly nudge. An example from Tracy's life is she often joins a local running club. Meeting new friends who have the same interests makes it easy to get out of bed early in the mornings to run while preparing for her next race.

Consider a coach to help in your health journey. Check out the Longevity Coaching Program on:

www.longevitycodes.com.

Conclusion

Need more incentive to start an exercise program? Here are a few additional benefits: it improves mood, helps with sleep, promotes good joint health, increases circulation, reduces the risk of breast and colon cancer, lowers stroke and heart disease, helps maintain an ideal body weight, and decreases the risk of developing Type 2 diabetes.

Start right now to get healthy! Don't wait for that health scare or next year but start today.

Discover your "WHY" for wanting to get healthy. Make sure the reason is for you and not because your doctor, family member, or friends want you to.

"You must find the activities you enjoy because if you enjoy it, you'll do it over and over again."
Tracy Herbert

Chapter 20
Accountability for Accelerated Results

How do you feel about being held accountable? Most people take that negatively, but is it? It goes against human nature because people do not want to relinquish perceived control to another person.

While your first thought might be unfavorable with the concept of an accountability partner, keep reading because this insight will change your viewpoint and strategies.

Here's why you must have the right accountability partner:

Motivate

An accountability partner helps to keep you motivated to achieve your goals. A key strategy to reach your goals is to tell others about it, which makes it more likely you will do it. The same is true, with an accountability partner. You permit them to ask the tough questions. When someone repeatedly asks about the status of your goal, it motivates you to keep the promises you made to yourself and them.

Cheerleader

When your willpower is low, your accountability partner will be your biggest cheerleader. Others see your strengths better than you do! They will be there to remind you that you can accomplish whatever you set out to do. A good cheerleader will be there every step of the way, saying, "Yes, you can, you can do this!"

Nudge

They help keep your goals at the top of mind. An accountability partner never allows you to put your big goals on the back burner and will continuously nudge you along the path.

Meet Deadlines

Accountability partners help meet deadlines. Remembering you committed to someone will help you stay on track. Otherwise, you might give yourself a pass and lose motivation to hit a goal by a specific date.

Corrections

An accountability partner helps to make mid-course corrections before you get too far off track. By frequently talking with your accountability partner, you can spot negative trends before they become obstacles too hard to overcome. They help you stay on track to meet your goal. When you have setbacks, your accountability partner enables you to get back on course.

The importance of having an accountability partner is evident, but how do you find the right person? It may not be your spouse or best friend, but look for someone who asks the difficult questions and has the right temperament to keep you accountable. This task is not for everyone. Choose wisely.

If you have tried in the past without success, you likely had the wrong person.

Here are a few things to ask yourself:

- Do I trust them to keep the discussions confidential?
- Are they good encouragers?
- Will they be honest and ask the tough questions?
- Can they hold my feet to the fire and not accept flimsy excuses?
- How likely will they invest the appropriate amount of time needed?
- Am I willing to be vulnerable and be held accountable?
- Will I make it a priority?

If you have difficulty finding the right person, contact Longevity Codes for help:

https://www.longevitycodes.com

High achievers find value in hiring coaches to hold them accountable and achieve their goals. We have found this to be true in our lives. Even though we are coaches, we invest a significant amount of money in coaches and accountability partners to keep us on track.

Think about the value of achieving your goal to be healthier and live longer. It is impossible to put a price on it!

Set goals, audacious or not, and create a system to achieve them.

www.LongevityCodes.com

The tool to help you achieve the next level is an accountability partner or coach. Remember the last time you started an exercise program? How long did you stick with the plan by yourself? When you have a friend checking in on you, you will do it!

Hopefully, you have people in your life to help you stay on track like we do.

"Accountability breeds response-ability."
Stephen Covey

Check out
LONGEVITY CODES COACHING PROGRAM
www.LongevityCodes.com
Our **Longevity Codes Certified Coach** will help you implement the principles in this book and provide the tools and accountability you need to achieve fast results.

www.LongevityCodes.com

Chapter 21

Sleep Better and Live Longer

If you are struggling with sleep, you are not alone. According to the Center for Disease Control[1], 35% of adults are not getting enough sleep.

Sleep issues are a real problem, especially as people age.

American Sleep Association reports[2]:

- 50-70 million U.S. adults suffer from sleep disorders
- 48% report snoring
- 37.9% reported unintentionally falling asleep during the day at least once in the preceding month
- 4.7% disclosed nodding off or falling asleep while driving at least once in the prior month
- Drowsy driving is responsible for 1,550 fatalities and 40,000 nonfatal injuries annually in the United States
- Insomnia is the most common specific sleep disorder, with short term issues reported by about 30% of adults and chronic insomnia by 10%
- 25 Million U.S. adults have obstructive sleep apnea

Want to know the sleep longevity connection?

Researchers studied[3] the sleep patterns of people over 85. The study concluded that poor sleep and sleep deprivation might cause inflammation, oxidative stress, mitochondrial decline, and cellular senescence, often called zombie cells. One of the common factors between the oldest participants in the study is they had good slow-wave sleep, which is the deepest stage of non-REM sleep. Another commonality was well-established sleep patterns and good HDL cholesterol levels. This study found a strong correlation between age-related diseases and chronic sleep restriction along with disruptions in the sleep-wake cycle.

Maiken Nedergaard, a University of Rochester neuroscientist, said sleep is "It's like a dishwasher that keeps flushing through to wash the dirt away." Without getting the quality sleep needed, your brain will not detox properly. Dr. Nedergaard's research points to the possibility of becoming susceptible to Alzheimer's as people age. The issue could be you are not flushing the molecular trash that builds up in your brain, which affects your cognitive ability.

Another factor to consider is a bodyweight connection and sleep. Sleep deprivation hurts the body's leptin and ghrelin production. The more ghrelin you produce, the more your body stimulates hunger, which causes the brain to tell you it's time to eat again, even if it's not. Leptin tells you it's time to stop eating, or in other words, it suppresses your appetite. No wonder all the experts are now realizing the importance of good sleep for weight loss and lowering the risk of developing Type 2 diabetes.

"Sleep: The golden chain that ties health and our bodies together."
Thomas Dekker

That is so true!!

The heavier you are, the more difficult it is to fall asleep and stay asleep. If you sleep too little or too much, it often causes you to eat more substantial portions of food. That could be the never-ending spiral that's extremely difficult to stop.

The right amount is critical. What's the right amount? It varies from person to person, but most research suggests getting about seven to eight hours of uninterrupted sleep is ideal.

The International Diabetes Federation suggests doctors who diagnose their patients with Type 2 diabetes be tested for sleep apnea and vice versa because they are closely related. A study[3] found that a substantial proportion of patients with Type 2 diabetes also suffer from Obstructive Sleep Apnea but often goes undiagnosed.

Another study[4] suggests that chronic sleep loss increases the risk of diabetes and obesity. It concluded that poor sleep affects glucose regulation, changes appetite, which causes overeating, and decreases energy. Participants in another study[5] had only five hours of sleep for seven days. They found it significantly reduced their insulin sensitivity. The correlation between the sustained periods of insufficient sleep and insulin resistance or Type 2 diabetes is concerning.

Struggling occasionally to get a good night's sleep is not the problem. Chronic sleep issues are the real concern. The exciting news is you can take steps to improve your sleep habits. Everyone is busy, but you must make sure that you allow yourself enough time to sleep. Do not use being swamped as an excuse!

Honestly, you need to set boundaries for yourself that helps you achieve a good night's sleep, not just time in bed. If you're lying in bed wide awake, it's not helping to repair your cells. After a restful night's sleep, you will feel more productive and even happier. When making sleep a priority, you are protecting your health today and in the future.

> *"Early to bed and early to rise makes a person healthy, wealthy, and wise."*
> Benjamin Franklin

Need to Get More Sleep?

- Go to bed and wake up at the same time every day. The difference should be no more than an hour, which helps your circadian rhythm.
- Spend the hour before bed in quiet time
- Avoid bright artificial light, like a TV, phone, or computer screen. Bright lights can motion the brain to wake up.
- Alcohol can wreak havoc. When drinking, choose early and not a late evening to help with sleep, for longevity and good health drink in moderation.
- Avoid heavy meals within a couple of hours of bedtime.
- Avoid caffeine after 2 PM because it stays in your system for eight hours. Remember, even drinking something healthy like green tea, yet though it has less caffeine than coffee, could still affect your sleep patterns.
- Exercise is imperative, but don't do anything strenuous an hour or so before bedtime. Yoga is fine.
- Getting outside and getting fresh air and sunshine is essential, especially for sleep.
- Keep your bedroom quiet and dark
- Take a warm bath
- Practice relaxation and deep breathing techniques

www.LongevityCodes.com

- Keep your bedroom cool. Some studies suggest keeping temperatures between 60 and 68 degrees are best for optimal sleep.
- Reduce stress levels
- Meditation helps
- Know your circadian rhythm. If you're naturally a night owl, don't try to force yourself to be an early bird.
- Krill Oil or other quality omega-3 fatty acids help improve sleep and helps to fall asleep faster.
- Magnesium can help some sleep deeper by lowering stress while regulating melatonin levels.

Melatonin is another supplement known to help with sleep. The problem is many take supplements at a much higher dose than the dose shown to be sufficient of .1 to .5 milligrams—another example where more is not better. Test melatonin supplementation to see what works best for you but start with a low dose.

Redox Signaling Molecules has dramatically improved our sleep. Tracy, who's postmenopausal, has been having sleep issues for years. Since using Redox Signaling Molecules, she is sleeping better now than she has in over 30 years, and especially since having kids.

To learn more about this breakthrough technology, go to: www.LongevityCodes.com/redox

As with everything, talk with your doctor first, especially adding supplements. If you're having sleep issues, discuss it with your physician first. Consider letting your doctor know you want to improve your sleep naturally, if possible. Most sleep medications have nasty side effects.

> *"A good laugh and a long sleep are the best cures in the doctor's book."*
> Irish Proverb

Need more reasons why you need to take control of your sleep?

- Cancer risks increase with lack of sleep such as breast, prostate, and colorectal cancer
- Immune system suffers
- It reduces sex drive
- More prone to accidents ---- three times greater risk of a car accident when you have less than six hours of sleep according to the National Sleep Foundation
- Lack of sleep raises the risk of heart disease
- Cognitive abilities suffer when sleep-deprived

In a study[6] of 21,268 twins for over 22 years, it found that getting less than seven or more than eight hours of sleep each night had an increased risk of death. The study found that short sleep (<7 hours) increased the risk of death for men 26% and women by 21%. But also concluded a risk from sleeping too long (>8 hours) had an increased risk of death by 24% for men and 17% for women. The study concluded the associations between sleep and mortality are complicated. Still, there is increased risk from both short and long sleep patterns.

It's evident that sleep is a critical longevity strategy, and if you're not getting between seven to eight hours of **high-quality** sleep, make this your focus. Your cellular health and longevity depend on it.

Chapter 22
Supplements for Longevity

Supplements are important!! This chapter will dig deeper to see how supplements improve health. Always check with your medical team before supplementing because it can cause adverse reactions to many medications. Don't feel like you must run out and buy all of these but reading this information will point you in the right direction.

Longevity starts with a focus on cellular health! The supplements covered in this chapter help support healthy cells.

The most important strategy is to keep away from things that hurt your cells and then replace them with something to protect them. Once your cells are protected, they have what is needed to thrive and function at their best.

At the time of this writing, these are our top 10 supplements but will always be changing because of research.

Here are the Longevity Secrets top 10 Supplement list

#1 - Redox Signaling Molecules

As covered in previous chapters, this Nobel Prize-winning scientific discovery is first on the list because so few have heard about this technology. Scientists are calling this the biggest health breakthrough since penicillin. Redox

Signaling Molecules help cells communicate and function better. The body loses its natural ability to produce these molecules about 10% per decade after puberty. Scientists have discovered how to create these molecules outside the body and stabilize them in a liquid and gel form. Drinking Redox Signaling Molecules and using the gel on the skin daily is our #1 longevity strategy. You can learn more about this breakthrough in Chapter 8 or follow this link: www.LongevityCodes.com/redox

#2 - Curcumin

A bright yellow color, this compound comes from the turmeric root. Many serious health conditions, including cancer, diabetes, heart disease, and Alzheimer's, are attributed to chronic inflammation. It would take a large amount of turmeric root in meals, but taking a curcumin supplement is the best way for the maximum impact on health and inflammation. Studies have shown that curcumin supplementation is as effective as over-the-counter pain relievers without the negative side effects. Learn more in Chapter 12 on reducing aches and pains associated with aging.

#3 - Essential Vitamins & Minerals

In today's environment of processed and packaged foods, it is difficult to get the vitamins and minerals needed for maximum health from foods. Most experts agree that only consuming organic foods, you still will not receive the nutrients you once did. Important nutrients are missing in the depleted soil. The vitamins mentioned in this book are high quality and not the type typically found in big-box stores. Economical vitamins are a waste of money and likely will not make it to a cellular level. Make sure to purchase a quality multivitamin that is well researched and has the forms that are best absorbed by your body. Key vitamins and minerals to focus on are magnesium, selenium, B-vitamins, and Vitamin E. Test your vitamin levels before purchasing to see if you are deficient. Your physician will help you review the results and design a regime that works best for you. The RDA is not the best strategy to follow since these are the minimum recommendations. The recommendations are enough to keep you from getting ill from a deficiency, and not focused on optimal health.

Of course, Vitamin C is one of the best antioxidants to take. Antioxidants are known to prevent free radical cell damage. Make sure you are getting enough Vitamin C.

There are critics that reference studies concluding that taking multivitamin supplements show no reduction in lowering the risk of heart disease, cancer, and cognitive decline. We question the quality of the multivitamin supplements used in the studies referenced but want to be transparent and share both sides. Some suggest you can get all the nutrients needed from eating a healthy balanced diet, but this is difficult for the reasons mentioned earlier. That would be the best option but difficult for optimal health. That's what this book is all about!

#4 - Fisetin

Fisetin is a fairly new supplement to come on the scene and has strong anti-inflammatory properties. It's a flavonoid that helps to slow aging and lengthen lifespan and healthspan.

Research is showing fisetin may improve brain health and memory. Promising research is showing it may protect against stroke, Alzheimer's, and depression symptoms. Strawberries have the largest concentration, but you would need to eat 37 a day. Supplementing may be a viable option.

#5 - Resveratrol

Polyphenols protect the body against cellular damage, and Resveratrol is a powerhouse. Cellular stress puts you at a higher risk for things like cancer and heart disease. It's often called the red wine molecule and is found it the skin of red grapes. While research is ongoing, the evidence is strong that it provides many health and longevity benefits. First, it's believed to help fight heart disease, cancer, Alzheimer's, diabetes, and of course, anti-aging. Be careful here if you're going to buy a supplement because many have more hype than help. Do your research and go with only the most reputable manufacturers.

There are other polyphenols to consider adding to your diet. Berries are all rich in polyphenols, along with dark chocolate, pomegranate, green tea, turmeric, ginger, and cinnamon.

Each day we mix a red blend of polyphenols in water. It tastes great and gives us a jump start on getting the antioxidants needed.

#6 - Collagen

The body's most abundant protein is collagen. It is the primary component of your skin, ligaments, muscles, tendons, and connective tissues. Collagen has been shown to help improve skin, relieve joint pain, improve heart health, prevent bone loss, gut health, and brain health. There are three types of collagen. Type I found in the skin, bones, teeth, tendons, and some connective tissues. Cartilage and eyes contain Type II. At the same time, Type III collagen is in your skin, along with muscles and blood vessels. Like many things, collagen degrades with age, which is why supplementation makes a lot of sense. Good food sources that help the body produce more collagen naturally are:

- Fish
- Red, dark green, and orange vegetables
- Citrus fruits
- Protein
- Beans
- Berries
- Garlic
- Flax seeds
- Avocados
- Soy

In our daily morning protein and green shake, we get extra collagen by adding bone broth. Purchasing high quality powered or capsules are best.

#7 - Coenzyme Q10

An essential anti-aging supplement to consider is also called CoQ10. One study[1] concluded that aging and chronic diseases might be related to low levels of CoQ10 in tissues and organs. Ubiquinol, which is the reduced form of CoQ10, is naturally occurring in the body and found in every cell.

www.LongevityCodes.com

Ubiquinol plays a role in 95 percent of the body's energy production, and its primary function is the synthesis of cellular energy. This enzyme decreases with age and oxidative stress and is in the inner mitochondrial membrane.

Research has shown that CoQ10 can help with: headaches, heart disease, skin health, diabetes, cancer prevention, brain health, and lung health.

Good food sources for CoQ10 are:

- Organ meats like the heart, liver, and kidney
- Pork, beef, and chicken
- Trout, herring, mackerel, and sardine
- In some vegetables such as spinach, cauliflower, and broccoli
- In fruits like oranges and strawberries
- In soybeans, lentils, and peanuts
- In nuts and seeds like pistachios and sesame seeds

Even if you consume higher quantities of these foods in your daily diet, you might want to consider supplementing to be sure you're getting enough CoQ10.

If you are on a statin drug for cholesterol, talk to your doctor about adding CoQ10 because this drug depletes it from your body.

Do your research. Enough said!

#8 - Omega-3 Fatty Acids

Omega-3's have a great deal of scientific evidence to support its health benefits. The two types of omega-3 fatty acids are eicosapentaenoic acid (EPA) and docosahexaenoic acid (DHA).

Here's a list of some of the known benefits of omega-3's:

- Fights depression and anxiety
- Fights inflammation
- Fights autoimmune diseases
- Good for the skin
- Promotes brain health during pregnancy and early life
- Improves heart disease risk factors
- Reduces symptoms of ADHD in children
- Improve mental disorders
- Fights age-related mental decline and Alzheimer's
- Improves eye health
- Cancer prevention
- Reduces asthma in children
- Reduces fatty liver
- Improves bone and joint health
- Improves sleep

Does that list encourage you to add omega-3's daily? If so, here are some healthy options:

- Salmon is an excellent source of omega-3's, and others are cold-water fatty fish, such as mackerel, tuna, herring, and sardines
- Nuts and seeds like flaxseed, chia seeds, and walnuts are also excellent sources
- Good plant sources are flaxseed oil, soybean oil, and canola oil

There are varying qualities of omega-3 supplements on the market. Choose wisely. One supplement that has been talked about recently is krill oil, and some researchers believe it's better than fish oil supplements. Krill oil is also rich in EPA and DHA's, and some studies suggest that bodies might absorb and use krill oil fatty acids better than fish oil. Some claim that krill oil is less likely to go rancid, which can be a problem with fish oil capsules. In our opinion, the evidence is strong enough to make it our first choice as an omega-3 supplement.

#9 - Probiotics

A staple in our daily health toolbox is probiotics. Fred has been taking probiotic supplements for over 20 years, and it has dramatically improved his health. Just like so many others! The gut is the primary source for the production of immune cells, which helps to fight off the harmful gut bacteria. Probiotics help with longevity because it effectively fights off infectious diseases, to help live longer.

Scientists at McGill University fed fruit flies a combination of probiotics and Triphala, which is an herbal supplement, and they lived 60% longer[2]. Triphala has been used in healing remedies for over 1,000 years. It's a staple in traditional India Ayurvedic medicine. It is an herbal concoction using three medicinal plants which are native to India, and each has their healing properties.

The gut has a combination of healthy bacteria and harmful or damaging bacteria. Creating a healthy gut environment encourages good bacteria to thrive. Years of overusing antibiotics have wreaked havoc on the good bacteria. Even though antibiotics save lives, it kills off the good guys while removing the harmful bacteria. If you have a bacterial infection that requires antibiotics, take probiotics to replace those getting killed off. Overprescribing antibiotics has been a problem that has serious ramifications. Super Bugs can become resistant, making it difficult to kill them.

To add more probiotics through food, choose yogurt, but watch out for added sugar. Other good choices of fermented foods are pickled vegetables, kombucha, kimchi, sauerkraut, miso, and kefir.

Here are some known benefits of probiotics and a healthy gut:

- Probiotics can help boost your immune system
- Boost "good" bacteria
- Improve some digestive disorders
- Some strains help with heart health
- Can improve some mental health disorders
- Prevent and treat diarrhea
- Improve athletic performance
- Reduce the severity of some allergies
- May help in weight loss and reduction of belly fat

#10 - Whey Protein

Whey protein has been proven beneficial for athletes and building muscles. Scientists are now showing it also has anti-aging properties.

Whey protein provides the liver amino acids needed to build glutathione, which is the body's master antioxidant. Glutathione helps your liver neutralize toxins found in foods, cells, and the environment. It supports the crucial mitochondria, which helps boost immunity.

Select cold-processed and grass-fed whey protein for best results. Heating whey during refinement can destroy nutrients that diminish its effectiveness.

Here are some of the potential health benefits of whey protein:

- Source of high-quality protein
- Lower blood pressure
- Helps with weight loss
- Promotes muscle growth
- Help treat Type 2 diabetes
- Beneficial in Inflammatory Bowel Disease
- Helps reduce inflammation
- Enhance the body's antioxidant defense
- Reduces hunger

Having too much protein in the diet has long been debated. The issues are related to an animal protein more than plant protein. A diet too high in protein can be unhealthy.

Find what works best for your body. Everyone is different, and what works for one may not work for someone else. Research and discover hidden gems to help you live a longer, healthier life. Always choose high-quality supplements and check with your doctor before taking them.

Get additional FREE RESOURCES at
www.LongevityCodes.com

www.LongevityCodes.com

Chapter 23
Age Slower with Longer Telomeres

Telomeres are critical for aging healthy and is a Greek word meaning <u>telos</u> "end" and <u>meros</u> "part." In other words, it is the end part of DNA.

Telomeres are like the plastic caps on the end of shoelaces. Without this coating, shoelaces would become frayed to the point they could no longer do their job. Your DNA needs these telomere caps to keep the strands from becoming damaged to the point where your cells are not functioning correctly.

Every cell in the body has DNA, which dictates how it replicates and the role it plays in the body. Skin cells, bone cells, heart cells, you name it, and it requires healthy DNA to duplicate accurately, which is why telomeres are so important.

When cells replicate, telomeres become shorter to the point where they are too short to do their job correctly, which causes cellular aging. Factors like stress, unhealthy diet, and other harmful habits can contribute to shortened telomeres. Telomere length signifies biological age, not chronological age.

Scientific studies show a strong correlation between cellular aging and short telomeres.

Scientists[1] compared the aging process in a variety of different species. Researchers concluded aging was determined by how quickly telomeres shrink in all life forms.

For example, humans have much shorter telomere lengths compared to mice, but humans have a much longer lifespan. Mice telomeres shorten 100 times faster than humans, and it's now believed this accelerated shortening is the real difference in longevity.

Bottom line, it appears the lifespan of all lifeforms are determined by how quickly telomeres shorten.

With this information, what can you do?

The answer is both simple and complex. The simple part is slowing down or stopping the shortening of your telomeres, and you could live longer. The complicated part is it's not that easy.

Follow these strategies to slow down the shortening of telomeres.

Lifestyle

A study[2] included men with a low risk of prostate cancer determined by a biopsy. In this study, the men separated into two groups; one being the "control group" and the other called the "intervention group." The men in the control group made no lifestyle changes. In contrast, the other group followed a lifestyle change program that included diet, stress management, physical activity, and social support. The study concluded the group adhering to the lifestyle changes had a significant improvement in telomere length compared to the group with no modifications.

This study is encouraging! Everything you do to improve cellular health will naturally help you keep longer and healthier telomeres.

www.LongevityCodes.com

Diet

Another study[3] stated that the aging process and age-related diseases are impacted by your nutrition, which might affect telomerase (an anti-aging enzyme) activity. It concluded that lifestyle and diet interventions could promote a longer lifespan but, more importantly, an increased healthspan.

Fiber

A diet rich in fiber may also help maintain telomere length. A research study[4] compared the fiber intake of 5,674 adults. Those with a high fiber diet had longer telomeres and had a biological age five years younger age than those who consumed low fiber diets. The study found people who ate large amounts of nuts and seeds tend to have longer telomeres than people who eat smaller amounts.

Other benefits of a high fiber diet include:

- Getting to and maintaining a healthy weight
- Lowers risk of Type 2 diabetes
- A natural detoxifier
- Lower the risk of heart disease
- Improves gut bacteria
- Reduces the risk of certain cancers

Diet is essential for having healthy and longer telomeres.

Physical Activity!

Want to add nine years to your biological age? A study[5] found that people living a physically active lifestyle had approximately a nine-year biological aging advantage over those living a sedentary life. It concluded it might be related to the longer telomeres of the physically active participants, which could explain the reduction in cellular aging.

Your biological age is more important than your chronological age.

Need a reason to get off the couch? A biological age that's nine years younger ought to be reason enough.

Chronic Stress

Chronic stress damages your health, but is it because of the adverse effects it has on telomeres? Excessive hormone levels of cortisol and epinephrine are linked[6] to shortened telomeres.

Researchers found[7] how stress impacts health by changing the rate of cellular aging. Women with high levels of stress had significantly higher oxidative stress, shorter telomeres, and lower telomerase activity. The low-stress women in the study had telomere lengths approximately ten years younger than the high-stress group. Stress can damage cells and promote age-related diseases much earlier in life.

Lengthening your telomeres is possible. What you want to avoid is shortening telomeres by making poor lifestyle choices. Practicing the health strategies found throughout this book will help you jumpstart your journey. Follow Tracy's 3M Formula – Mind-Mouth-Move to get started!

- **Mind** – Stress negatively impacts telomeres length
- **Mouth** – Food choices can either help or hurt telomeres
- **Move** – Physical activity improves telomere length

www.LongevityCodes.com

To avoid reducing telomere length, don't smoke, get good quality sleep, stay away from pollution as much as possible, and limit exposure to industrial chemicals.

Check out
LONGEVITY CODES COACHING PROGRAM
www.LongevityCodes.com
Our **Longevity Codes Certified Coach** will help you implement the principles in this book and provide the tools and accountability you need to achieve fast results.

Chapter 24
Don't Go It Alone

This book has provided you a wealth of information about living a longer, healthier life. The scientific studies and data on longevity continue. Amid all this information, people have questions about what is relevant to them and what information is trustworthy. People are often unclear on how they should get started, and how to deal effectively with setbacks and challenges.

Coaches play an important role in helping people achieve their goals. Professional athletes, executives, high achievers, and people wanting a better life find value in having a coach to help them achieve their goals.

The Role of a Coach

Here are vital roles a coach provides to help you achieve your goals:

Provide Specific Expertise

A Longevity Coach helps determine the information and practices needed. They guide you along the way by helping you implement the right strategies for your unique situation. Your coach has knowledge of anti-aging and health sciences that applies to your specific needs. This unique program is designed for you and will be your guide throughout the journey.

Discover Your WHY

One of the first ways your coach will help you is by discovering the "WHY" behind your need for change. When faced with setbacks, it is easy to lose sight of the motivation for change. When this happens, and it will, your coach will point you back to your "WHY" and help you overcome the obstacles.

Your Advocate

Your coach is here to guide, train, encourage, and motivate you towards results. With nonjudgmental encouragement, your coach will help you stay committed to making choices that best fit the results you expect. They will ask the right questions, be an active listener, point you in the right direction, and help find the best strategies.

Create A Customized Longevity Strategy

Do you know what is needed? The Longevity Strategy is designed specifically for you and helps to determine what's most important.

Accountability

After establishing the health plans and longevity goals, your coach will continue to guide you and hold you accountable every step of the way. If you have a friend or family member willing to help, ask them. Make sure they are prepared to ask the difficult questions and have the right temperament to keep you accountable. This role is not for everyone. A coach

www.LongevityCodes.com

is a partner to guide and help you make appropriate lifestyle choices.

Challenge

A good coach will cheer for you, keep you accountable, and challenge you to exceed the limits in a healthy way. After reaching your first milestone, they will challenge you to set even bigger goals while helping you reach them.

What you should look for in a Longevity Coach:

- ☑ Understands Longevity Codes key concepts
- ☑ Proven expertise in health and wellness
- ☑ Decades of coaching and implementing health strategies
- ☑ Practices what they preach
- ☑ Has excellent communication skills
- ☑ Provides applicable information that meets your unique style
- ☑ Not your friend, but someone who can help you reach your health goals
- ☑ Is an accountability partner
- ☑ Understands the value of team effort and allows you to explore ways to be successful
- ☑ Provides valuable and accurate information
- ☑ Helps you identify your "WHY" and understands what you are trying to accomplish
- ☑ Is excited and passionate for your personal growth
- ☑ Enables you to focus on today and the future
- ☑ Asks for and expects a commitment
- ☑ Is an active listener
- ☑ Can empathize with your unique situation

www.LongevityCodes.com

- ☑ Is the right fit with regards to personality
- ☑ Puts you at ease
- ☑ Seeks information by asking pertinent questions
- ☑ Allows you to do the work by setting goals
- ☑ Is passionate and knowledgeable about the health goals you are trying to reach

You are not alone! Take a deep breath, and remember it is NEVER too late.

"Everybody dies, but not everybody lives."
A Sachs

Check out
LONGEVITY CODES COACHING PROGRAM
www.LongevityCodes.com
Our **Longevity Codes Certified Coach** will help you implement the principles in this book and provide the tools and accountability you need to achieve fast results.

www.LongevityCodes.com

Chapter 25

What's Next?

The quest to understand how to live a longer and healthier life is a continuous process. Scientists and researchers discover new strategies daily to improve cellular health, how cells work, and optimize them effectively.

You may feel overwhelmed by all the information found in this book. If this is you, go to the Longevity Codes website, where you will find free resources along with opportunities to find additional support. No one should do this alone!

If you feel like you've been drinking out of a fire hose, pick one tactic found in this book and start now. Implementing too many changes at the same time only leads to failure. After mastering the first strategy, pick another and repeat the process while continuing with the first one. It's like interest; the compound effect over time leads to significant results.

Little steps equal big changes over time. Longevity is a marathon and not a sprint!

Adding quantity and quality for your life is the mission of this book.

SIX-F's

Following the approaches found in this book to improve health and longevity is an investment that pays enormous dividends. The payout in those extra years is what we call the SIX-F's.

www.LongevityCodes.com

Family

Spending more time with your spouse, kids, grandkids, and great-grandkids is an opportunity to impact more lives, bring joy, and leave a legacy.

Friends

The longest living people in the world have strong social support and spend time in the community with good friends.

Freedom

No one wants to be a burden on their families! What does freedom look like for you? For us, we want the ability to travel and not be stuck in a rocking chair.

Fun

Who does not want to have fun? When you practice strategies found in this book, living longer and heathier allows time to enjoy hobbies, have adventures, or play games with your grandchildren.

Fit

Our mentors played a significant role without even knowing it. At 86 and 84, they were able to hike to the bottom of the Grand Canyon. That may seem extreme, but having the right level of fitness allowed them to reach their goals. What does adding extra years of good health and an improved fitness level enable you to achieve?

Fulfillment

Now that you know how to add additional years to your life, spend those years fulfilling your purpose. What legacy do you want to leave?

The SIX-F's is what *Longevity Codes* is all about. Will the effort be worth it? You bet! Show the research found in this book to your doctor and work closely with him or her before implementing it.

Even though this is the end of the book, it's not the end of the journey.

Resources:

Listen to the weekly **Longevity Codes** podcast on all major podcast platforms.

Download the latest free resource at: https://www.longevitycodes.com/

Here's to you and your journey!

Fred and Tracy Herbert

www.LongevityCodes.com

Chapter 26

References

Chapter 1 - Foundational Approach to Longevity

None

Chapter 2 - Aging Paradigm Shift

(1) United Nations, World Population Prospects 2019: Data Booklet, Retrieved from https://population.un.org/wpp/Publications/Files/WPP2019_DataBooklet.pdf

(2) List of world records in masters athletics, (n.d.) In *Wikipedia*, retrieved February 1, 2020, from https://en.wikipedia.org/wiki/List_of_world_records_in_masters_athletics

Chapter 3 - Lessons from the Oldest Living People

(1) Dan Buettner, Sam Skemp, (2016, Jul 7), Blue Zones Lessons From the World's Longest Lived, Retrived from https://www.ncbi.nlm.nih.gov/pmc/articles/PMC6125071/

(2) Harvard Men's Health Watch, (2019, June 5, Revised), Marriage and men's health, Retrieved from https://www.health.harvard.edu/mens-health/marriage-and-mens-health

(3) Fatih Ozbay, MD, Douglas C. Johnson, PhD, Eleni Dimoulas, PhD, C.A. Morgan III, MD, MA, Dennis Charney, MD, and Steven Southwick, MD, (2007, May), Retrieved from https://www.ncbi.nlm.nih.gov/pmc/articles/PMC2921311/

Chapter 4 - The Motivation Factor

(1) Center for Disease Control and Prevention, (n.d.), Adult Obesity Facts, Retrieved from https://www.cdc.gov/obesity/data/adult.html

Chapter 5 - Prevention Principal

(1) Center for Disease Control and Prevention, (n.d.), About Chronic Diseases, Retrieved from https://www.cdc.gov/chronicdisease/about/index.htm
(2) Dr. Andrew Weil, (2013, March 10), U.S. manages disease, not health, Retrieved from https://www.cnn.com/2013/03/08/opinion/weil-health-care/index.html

Chapter 6 – The 3M Formula for Longer Life

(1) Jennifer Warner, (2005, June 15), Strong Friendships May Help You Live Longer, Retrieved from https://www.webmd.com/balance/news/20050615/strong-friendships-may-help-you-live-longer
(2) Department of Health and Human Services, (n.d.), Dietary Guidelines for Americans 2015*2020 Eighth Edition, Retrieved from https://health.gov/our-work/food-nutrition/2015-2020-dietary-guidelines/guidelines/appendix-1/
(3) Center for Disease Control and Prevention, (n.d.), Exercise or Physical Activity, Retrieved from https://www.cdc.gov/nchs/fastats/exercise.htm

Chapter 7 - Finding the Perfect Diet

(1) Mahmoud Abdelaal, Carel W. le Roux, Neil G. Docherty, (2017, April 5), Morbidity And Mortality Associated With Obesity, Retrieved from https://www.ncbi.nlm.nih.gov/pmc/articles/PMC5401682/

www.LongevityCodes.com

Chapter 8 - Critical Cell Signaling

(1) Bayani Uttara, Ajay V. Singh, Paolo Zamboni, R.T Mahajan, (2009, March 7) Oxidative Stress and Neurodegenerative Diseases: A Review of Upstream and Downstream Antioxidant Therapeutic Options, Retrieved from https://www.ncbi.nlm.nih.gov/pmc/articles/PMC2724665/

(2) American Autoimmune Related Diseases Association, (2018, September 17), Misconceptions about Autoimmune Diseases Still Exist, Retrieved from https://www.aarda.org/misconceptions-autoimmune-diseases-still-exist/

(3) Center for Disease Control, (n.d.), Arthritis, Retrieved from https://www.cdc.gov/chronicdisease/resources/publications/factsheets/arthritis.htm

(4) Center for Disease Control, (n.d.) Heart Disease Facts, Retrieved from https://www.cdc.gov/heartdisease/facts.htm

(5) Christopher V Almario, Megana L Ballal, William D Chey, Carl Nordstrom, Dinesh Khanna, Brennan M R Spiegel, (2018, Octover 15) Burden of Gastrointestinal Symptoms in the United States: Results of a Nationally Representative Survey of Over 71,000 Americans, Retrieved from https://www.ncbi.nlm.nih.gov/pmc/articles/PMC6453579/

Chapter 9 - Reversing Your Biological Age

(1) National Institutes of Health, (2014, July 8), NIH study finds extreme obesity may shorten life expectancy up to 14 years, Retrieved from https://www.wvdhhr.org/bph/oehp/obesity/mortality.htm

(2) Marta Jackowska, Mark Hamer, Livia A. Carvalho, Jorge D. Erusalimsky, Lee Butcher, Andrew Steptoe, (2012, October 29), Short Sleep Duration Is Associated with Shorter Telomere Length in Healthy Men: Findings from the Whitehall II Cohort Study,

www.LongevityCodes.com

https://journals.plos.org/plosone/article?id=10.1371/journal.pone.0047292

Chapter 10 – Beat Stress for Better Health

(1) National Institute of Mental Health. (n.d.), 5 Things You Should Know About Stress, Retrieved from https://www.nimh.nih.gov/health/publications/stress/index.shtml#pub3

(2) Epel ES, (2009, Jan-Mar), Psychological and Metabolic Stress: A Recipe for Accelerated Cellular Aging?, Retrieved from http://www.hormones.gr/503/article/psychological-and-metabolic-stress:-a-recipe%E2%80%A6.html

(3) Gail Matthews, PhD, (n.d.), Goals Research Summary, Retrieved from https://www.dominican.edu/directory-people/gail-matthews

Chapter 11 - Build a Strong Immune System

(1) Jennifer N. Morey, Ian A. Boggero, April B. Scott, Suzanne C. Segerstrom, (2015, October 1), Current Directions in Stress and Human Immune Function, Retrieved from https://www.ncbi.nlm.nih.gov/pmc/articles/PMC4465119/

(2) Michael R. Irwin, MD, (2012, August 1), Sleep and Infectious Disease Risk, Retrieved from https://www.ncbi.nlm.nih.gov/pmc/articles/PMC3397805/

(3) Michael Gleeson, (2016, September 26), Effects of exercise on immune function and risk of infection, Retrieved from https://www.mysportscience.com/single-post/2016/09/25/Strategies-to-reduce-illness-risk-in-athletes-Part-1-Behavioural-lifestyle-and-medical-strategies

(4) Veronica Lazar, Lia-Mara Ditu, Gratiela Gradisteanu Pircalabioru, Irina Gheorghe, Carmen Curutiu, Alina Maria Holban, Ariana Picu, Laura Petcu, Mariana Carmen Chifiriuc, (2018, Aug 15). Aspects of Gut Microbiota and Immune System Interactions in Infectious Diseases, Immunopathology, and Cancer, Retrieved from https://www.ncbi.nlm.nih.gov/pmc/articles/PMC6104162/

www.LongevityCodes.com

Chapter 12 - Eliminate Aches and Pains

(1) VA Office of Public and Intergovernmental Affairs, (2002, July 10), VA Study Questions Common Knee Surgery, Retrieved from https://www.va.gov/opa/pressrel/pressrelease.cfm?id=476

(2) National Council on Aging, (n.d.), Falls Prevention Facts. Retrieved from https://www.ncoa.org/news/resources-for-reporters/get-the-facts/falls-prevention-facts/

(3) Luigi Ferrucci1, Elisa Fabbri, (2018, September 20), Inflammageing: chronic inflammation in ageing, cardiovascular disease, and frailty, Retrieved from https://www.ncbi.nlm.nih.gov/pmc/articles/PMC6146930/

(4) Qiushan Tao, MD, Ting Fang Alvin Ang, MD, Charles DeCarli, MD, Sanford H. Auerbach, MD, Sheral Devine, PhD, Thor D. Stein, MD, PhD, Xiaoling Zhang, PhD, Joseph Massaro, PhD, Rhoda Au, PhD, Wei Qiao Qiu, MD, PhD, (2018, October 19), Association of Chronic Low-grade Inflammation With Risk of Alzheimer Disease in ApoE4 Carriers, Retrieved from https://www.ncbi.nlm.nih.gov/pmc/articles/PMC6324596/

Chapter 13 - Overcoming Setbacks

None

Chapter 14 - The Secret to More Energy

(1) Akbar M, Essa MM, Daradkeh 3, Abdelmegeed MA, Choi Y, Mahmood L, Song BJ, (2019, April 15), Mitochondrial dysfunction and cell death in neurodegenerative diseases through nitroxidative stress, Retrieved from https://www.ncbi.nlm.nih.gov/pubmed/26883165

Chapter 15 - Strategies for Better Gut Health

(1) Elena Biagi, Claudio Franceschi, Simone Rampelli, Marco Severgnini, Rita Ostan, Silvia Turroni, Clarissa Consolandi,

www.LongevityCodes.com

Sara Quercia, Maria Scurti, Daniela Monti, Miriam Capri, Patrizia Brigidi, Marco Candela, (2016, May 12),Gut Microbiota and Extreme Longevity, Retrieved from https://www.cell.com/current-biology/pdf/S0960-9822(16)30338-4.pdf

(2) Center for Disease Control and Prevention, (n.d.), Antibiotic Prescribing and Use in the U.S., Retrieved from https://www.cdc.gov/antibiotic-use/stewardship-report/index.html

Chapter 16 – Taking Control of Your Health

(1) National Institute of Mental Health. (n.d.), 5 Things You Should Know About Wang, D B Dubal, (2015, June 16), Longevity factor klotho and chronic psychological stress, Retrieved from https://www.nature.com/articles/tp201581

Chapter 17 - The Master Antioxidant

(1) Gabriele Pizzino, Natasha Irrera, Mariapaola Cucinotta, Giovanni Pallio, Federica Mannino, Vincenzo Arcoraci, Francesco Squadrito, Domenica Altavilla, Alessandra Bitto,(2017, July 27), Oxidative Stress: Harms and Benefits for Human Health, Retrieved from https://www.hindawi.com/journals/omcl/2017/8416763/

(2) Vishwanath Venketaraman, Yaswant K. Dayaram, Meliza T. Talaue, and Nancy D. Connell1, (2005 March), Glutathione and Nitrosoglutathione in Macrophage Defense against Mycobacterium tuberculosis, Retrieved from https://www.ncbi.nlm.nih.gov/pmc/articles/PMC1064956/

(3) (World Health Organization, (2020, March 24), Tuberculosis, Retrieved from https://www.who.int/news-room/fact-sheets/detail/tuberculosis

(4) Flaim C, Kob M, Di Pierro, Herrmann, Lucchin,(2017, May 20), Effects of a whey protein supplementation on oxidative stress, body composition and glucose metabolism among overweight people affected by diabetes mellitus or impaired

fasting glucose: A pilot study, Retrieved from https://www.ncbi.nlm.nih.gov/pubmed/29053995
(5) Lenton KJ, Sané AT, Therriault H, Cantin AM, Payette H, Wagner JR., (2003, January 1), Vitamin C augments lymphocyte glutathione in subjects with ascorbate deficiency, Retrieved from https://www.ncbi.nlm.nih.gov/pubmed/12499341
(6) Johnston CS1, Meyer CG, Srilakshmi JC, (1993, July 1), Vitamin C elevates red blood cell glutathione in healthy adults, Retrieved from https://www.ncbi.nlm.nih.gov/pubmed/8317379
(7) Donatus IA1, Sardjoko, Vermeulen NP, (1990, June 15), Cytotoxic and cytoprotective activities of curcumin: Effects on paracetamol-induced cytotoxicity, lipid peroxidation and glutathione depletion in rat hepatocytes, Retrieved from https://www.ncbi.nlm.nih.gov/pubmed/2353930
(8) Elokda AS, Nielsen DH, (2007, October 1), Effects of exercise training on the glutathione antioxidant system, Retrieved from https://www.ncbi.nlm.nih.gov/pubmed/17925621
(9) Gambelunghe C, Rossi R, Micheletti A, Mariucci G, Rufini S, (2001 March 1), Physical exercise intensity can be related to plasma glutathione levels, Retrieved from https://www.ncbi.nlm.nih.gov/pubmed/11579999
(10) Joshi PC, Guidot DM, (2007, Jan 12), The alcoholic lung: epidemiology, pathophysiology, and potential therapies, Retrieved from https://www.ncbi.nlm.nih.gov/pubmed/17220370
(11) Gulec M, Ozkol H, Selvi Y, Tuluce Y, Aydin A, Besiroglu L, Ozdemir PG, (2012, February 28), Oxidative stress in patients with primary insomnia, Retrieved from https://www.ncbi.nlm.nih.gov/pubmed/22401887

Chapter 18 – Save Money While Living Longer

(1) The Nobel Prize in Physiology or Medicine, (2016, October 3), Retrieved from https://www.nobelprize.org/prizes/medicine/2016/press-release/
(2) Min Wei, Sebastian Brandhorst, Mahshid Shelehchi, Hamed Mirzaei, Chia Wei Cheng, Julia Budniak, Susan Groshen,

Wendy J. Mack, Esra Guen, Stefano Di Biase, Pinchas Cohen, Todd E. Morgan, Tanya Dorff, Kurt Hong, Andreas Michalsen, Alessandro Laviano, Valter D. Longo, (2017, October 28), Fasting-mimicking diet and markers/risk factors for aging, diabetes, cancer, and cardiovascular disease, Retrieved from
https://www.ncbi.nlm.nih.gov/pmc/articles/PMC6816332/

Chapter 19 - Move for Life

(1) NHSUK, (2018, February 20), Light activity 'may be enough to help you live longer', Retrieved from https://www.nhs.uk/news/lifestyle-and-exercise/light-activity-may-be-enough-help-you-live-longer/

(2) Zhao M, Veeranki SP, Li S, Steffen LM, Xi B, (2019, March 19), Beneficial associations of low and large doses of leisure time physical activity with all-cause, cardiovascular disease and cancer mortality: a national cohort study of 88,140 US adults, Retrieved from https://www.ncbi.nlm.nih.gov/pubmed/30890520

(3) Hildebrand JS, Gapstur SM, Campbell PT, Gaudet MM, Patel AV, (2013, October 22), Recreational physical activity and leisure-time sitting in relation to postmenopausal breast cancer risk., Retrieved from https://www.ncbi.nlm.nih.gov/pubmed/24097200

(4) American Diabetes Association, (n.d.), Blood Sugar and Exercise, Retrieved from https://www.diabetes.org/fitness/get-and-stay-fit/getting-started-safely/blood-glucose-and-exercise

(5) W W Tigbe, M H Granat, N Sattar, M E J Lean, (2017, January 31), time spent in sedentary posture is associated with waist circumference and cardiovascular risk, Retrieved from https://www.ncbi.nlm.nih.gov/pubmed/28138134

(6) Kraschnewski JL, Sciamanna CN, Poger JM, Rovniak LS, Lehman EB, Cooper AB, Ballentine NH, Ciccolo JT, (2016, February 24), Is strength training associated with mortality benefits? A 15year cohort study of US older adults, Retrieved from https://www.ncbi.nlm.nih.gov/pubmed/26921660

www.LongevityCodes.com

Chapter 20 - Accountability for Accelerated Results

Longevity Codes for help. https://www.longevitycodes.com

Chapter 21 – Sleep Better and Live Longer

(1) Center for Disease Control and Prevention, (n.d.), Sleep and Sleep Disorders, Retrieved from https://www.cdc.gov/sleep/data_statistics.html
(2) American Sleep Association, (n.d.), Sleep and Sleep Disorder Statistics, Retrieved from https://www.sleepassociation.org/about-sleep/sleep-statistics/
(3) Sushmita Pamidi1, Esra Tasali, (2012, August 13), Obstructive Sleep Apnea and Type 2 Diabetes: Is There a Link?, Retrieved from https://www.ncbi.nlm.nih.gov/pmc/articles/PMC3449487/
(4) Kristen L. Knutsona, Eve Van Cauterbhttps, (2015, April 13), Associations between sleep loss and increased risk of obesity and diabetes, Retrieved from https://www.ncbi.nlm.nih.gov/pmc/articles/PMC4394987/
(5) Orfeu M. Buxton, Milena Pavlova, Emily W. Reid, Wei Wang, Donald C. Simonson, and Gail K. Adler1, (2010, June 28), ep Restriction for 1 Week Reduces Insulin Sensitivity in Healthy Men, Retrieved from https://www.ncbi.nlm.nih.gov/pmc/articles/PMC2927933/
(6) Christer Hublin, MD, PhD, Markku Partinen, MD, PhD, Markku Koskenvuo, MD, PhD, Jaakko Kaprio, MD, PhD, (2007, October 1), Sleep and Mortality: A Population-Based 22-Year Follow-Up Study, Retrieved from https://academic.oup.com/sleep/article/30/10/1245/2696836

Chapter 22 - Supplements for Longevity

(1) Juan D. Hernández-Camacho, Michel Bernier, Guillermo López-Lluch and Plácido Navas, (2018, February 5), Coenzyme Q10 Supplementation in Aging and Disease, Retrieved from https://www.ncbi.nlm.nih.gov/pmc/articles/PMC5807419/

www.LongevityCodes.com

(2) Susan Westfall, Nikita Lomis, Satya Prakash, (2018, May 30), Longevity extension in Drosophila through gut-brain communication, Retrieved from https://www.nature.com/articles/s41598-018-25382-z

Chapter 23 - Age Slower with Longer Telomeres

(1) Kurt Whittemore, Elsa Vera, Eva Martínez-Nevado, Carola Sanpera, Maria A. Blasco, (2019, July 23), Telomere shortening rate predicts species life span, Retrieved from https://www.pnas.org/content/116/30/15122
(2) Dean Ornish, MD, Jue Lin, PhD, Prof June M Chan, PhD, Elissa Epel, PhD, Colleen Kemp, RN, Prof Gerdi Weidner, PhD, Ruth Marlin, MD, Steven J Frenda, MA, Mark Jesus M Magbanua, PhD, Jennifer Daubenmier, PhD, PhD, Nancy K Hills, PhD, Nita Chainani-Wu, DMD, Prof Peter R Carroll, MD, Elizabeth H Blackburn, PhD, (2013, October 1), Effect of comprehensive lifestyle changes on telomerase activity and telomere length in men with biopsy-proven low-risk prostate cancer: 5-year follow-up of a descriptive pilot study, Retrieved from https://www.thelancet.com/journals/lanonc/article/PIIS1470-2045%2813%2970366-8/fulltext#
(3) Virginia Boccardi, Giuseppe Paolisso, and Patrizia Mecocci, (2016, January 8), Nutrition and lifestyle in healthy aging: the telomerase challenge, Retrieved from https://www.ncbi.nlm.nih.gov/pmc/articles/PMC4761710/
(4) Larry A. Tucker, (2018, March 23), Dietary Fiber and Telomere Length in 5674 U.S. Adults: An NHANES Study of Biological Aging, Retrieved from https://www.ncbi.nlm.nih.gov/pmc/articles/PMC5946185/#__ffn_sectitle
(5) Larry A Tucker, (2017, July), Physical Activity and Telomere Length in U.S. Men and Women: An NHANES Investigation, Retrieved from https://www.ncbi.nlm.nih.gov/pubmed/28450121
(6) Eleanor Law, Afaf Girgis, Sylvie Lambert, Lambert Sylvie, Janelle Levesque, Hilda Pickett, (2016, April-June), Telomeres and Stress: Promising Avenues for Research in

Psycho-Oncology, Retrieved from https://pubmed.ncbi.nlm.nih.gov/27981152-telomeres-and-stress-promising-avenues-for-research-in-psycho-oncology/

(7) Elissa S Epel, Elizabeth H Blackburn, Jue Lin, Firdaus S Dhabhar, Nancy E Adler, Jason D Morrow, Richard M Cawthon, (2004, December 7), Accelerated Telomere Shortening in Response to Life Stress, Retrieved from https://pubmed.ncbi.nlm.nih.gov/15574496-accelerated-telomere-shortening-in-response-to-life-stress/

Chapter 24 - **Don't Go It Alone**

Learn more about the Longevity Codes Coaching Program:
https://www.longevitycodes.com

Chapter 25 – **What's Next?**

Learn more and get free resources at:
https://www.longevitycodes.com

www.LongevityCodes.com

Connect with Us

Below are links on how you can connect with us.

Fred Herbert
Email: Fred@FredHerbert.com
Longevity Codes website:
www.LongevityCodes.com
Lean about Redox Signaling Molecules:
www.LongevityCodes.com/redox

Tracy Herbert
Email: Tracy@TracyHerbert.com
Website: www.TracyHerbert.com
Your Diabetes Breakthrough Podcast
www.YourDiabetesBreakthrough.com
Bring Tracy in as a speaker for your next event:
www.TracyHerbert.com/speaker

Check out
LONGEVITY CODES COACHING PROGRAM
www.LongevityCodes.com
Our **Longevity Codes Certified Coach** will help you implement the principles in this book and provide the tools and accountability you need to achieve fast results.

Get additional FREE RESOURCES at
www.LongevityCodes.com

Made in the USA
Middletown, DE
30 June 2020